JAN

CW00926928

Regarded by Augusto Boal as the international icon of his vision, Jana Sanskriti are the leading practitioners of Theatre of the Oppressed and Forum Theatre in India and the East.

The group has worked continuously with rural communities in West Bengal since its beginnings in 1985 to reconfigure social and political relationships through theatre, achieving both a solid regional presence and an international reputation.

This book combines:

- a biography of the group, charting their history, methodology and modes of operation
- an examination of Jana Sanskriti through the writings of their founder, Sanjoy Ganguly
- a detailed analysis of their performance events and practices, including the plays collected in Ganguly's *Where We Stand* (2009)
- practical exercises and games, taken from Jana Sanskriti's workshops and festivals.

As a first step towards critical understanding, and as an initial exploration before going on to further, primary research, *Routledge Performance Practitioners* offer unbeatable value for today's student.

Ralph Yarrow is Emeritus Professor of Drama and Comparative Literature at the University of East Anglia, UK.

ROUTLEDGE PERFORMANCE PRACTITIONERS

Series editors: Franc Chamberlain and Bernadette Sweeney

'Small, neat (handbag sized!) volumes; a good mix of theory and practice, written in a refreshingly straightforward and informative style ... *Routledge Performance Practitioners* are good value, easy to carry around, and contain all the key information on each practitioner – a perfect choice for the student who wants to get a grip on the big names in performance from the past hundred years.' - *Total Theatre*

Routledge Performance Practitioners is an innovative series of introductory handbooks on key figures in contemporary performance practice.

Each volume focuses on a theatre-maker who has transformed the way we understand theatre and performance. The books are carefully structured to enable the reader to gain a good grasp of the fundamental elements underpinning each practitioner's work. They provide an inspiring springboard for students on twentieth century, contemporary theatre, and theatre history courses.

Now revised and reissued, these compact, well-illustrated and clearly written books unravel the contribution of modern theatre's most charismatic innovators, through:

- personal biography
- explanation of key writings
- description of significant productions
- reproduction of practical exercises.

Volumes currently available in this series:

For more information about this series, please visit: https://www.routledge.com/Routledge-Performance-Practitioners/book-series/RPP

JANA SANSKRITI

Performance as a New Politics

Ralph Yarrow

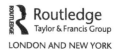

Routledge
Taylor & Francis Group

LONDON AND NEW YORK

First published 2022
by Routledge
2 Park Square, Milton Park, Abingdon, Oxon OX14 4RN

and by Routledge
605 Third Avenue, New York, NY 10158

Routledge is an imprint of the Taylor & Francis Group, an informa business

British Library Cataloguing-in-Publication Data
A catalogue record for this book is available from the British Library

Library of Congress Cataloging-in-Publication Data
A catalog record has been requested for this book

ISBN: 978-0-367-25628-9 (hbk)
ISBN: 978-0-367-25629-6 (pbk)
ISBN: 978-0-429-28875-3 (ebk)

DOI: 10.4324/9780429288753

Typeset in Perpetua
by codeMantra

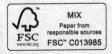

MIX
Paper from
responsible sources
FSC® C013985
www.fsc.org

Printed in the United Kingdom
by Henry Ling Limited

CONTENTS

FIGURES

EPIGRAPHS

'Brecht said "mixing one's wine may be a mistake but the old and new wisdom mix admirably". This is a good time to introspect what can we bring into our theatre, what is missing there, what are the strengths of our theatre. Theatre of the Oppressed is essentially dynamic and it has left spaces to hold new things. This is the time to develop that understanding.'

(Sanjoy Ganguly)

'We script intellectual power on stage that breaks the passivity within actors and spect-actors and turns them into Spect-Activists and Activists off stage respectively.'

(Sanjoy Ganguly)

FRONTISPIECES

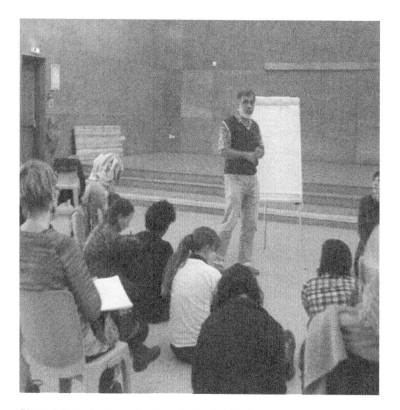

Figure 0.1 Sanjoy Ganguly at a workshop in Lille, France, 2013.

Photo: Jana Sanskriti

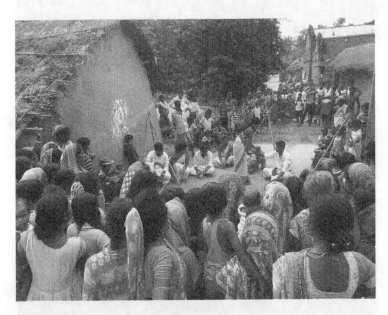

Figure 0.2 Jana Sanskriti rural performance, 2019, Purulia, West Bengal, India.

Photo: Jana Sanskriti

ACKNOWLEDGEMENTS

Many thanks to the Editors, Franc Chamberlain and Bernadette Sweeney, for thorough and precise comments. Thanks to Routledge for in-house editorial and processing.

For 20 years of interaction and exchange, guidance, assistance, logistics, openness to inspection, debate and participation in activities of many kinds, with a grace and generosity beyond compare, this book and its author owe an enormous debt to Jana Sanskriti, in all its facets and as all its members; and most of all to the central team members, the administrative team, and to Sima and Sanjoy Ganguly.

Thanks to Jana Sanskriti for permission to use all photographs in the book, with the exception of Fig. 6, Chapter One. Copyright remains with Jana Sanskriti.

Diagrams in Chapter Three by Shibsankar Bhattacharya, reproduced by permission of Jana Sanskriti.

Diagrams in Chapter Four and Fig. 7 in Chapter One by Zorya Yarrow.

ACKNOWLEDGEMENTS

A NOTE ON BENGALI PRONUNCIATION

- an initial 's' is pronounced 'sh': 'Sima' = Shima (i and ee are more or less interchangeable)
- a short 'a' is pronounced more like 'o': Bengali speakers call Sanjoy 'Shonjoy'
- in much of India the name is pronounced as 'Sanjay'
- 'Natak' – performance or play – is pronounced 'Natok'. Chittaranjan is called Chitta for short and is pronounced 'Chitto'; Satyaranjan is Satya for short, which is pronounced 'Shoto'; Kavita = 'Kovita'
- b and v are often interchangeable, as in Bhavan (building), which in Bengali spelling is 'Bhabhan'

WHO, WHAT, WHERE, WHY?

Jana Sanskriti's history, context and goals

INITIAL QUESTIONS

Why is Jana Sanskriti important? What can theatre practice and theatre practitioners learn from its work?

Jana Sanskriti (hereafter JS), founded in 1985 by Sanjoy Ganguly, is one of the best-known, and probably the largest and longest-lasting, Theatre of the Oppressed operations in the world. Theatre of the Oppressed (TO), created by Augusto Boal in the 1970s in Latin America, uses theatre practice to enable marginalised, disadvantaged and oppressed groups, communities and movements to analyse and confront the conditions they experience.

Jana Sanskriti means 'the people's culture'. Specifically, its remit is to create theatre *with* the people – mostly rural agricultural communities in West Bengal, India – as a means to address political, social and community issues in their everyday lives. What that means in practice is making plays which reflect those issues, using a form of theatre which enables members of the community to participate in the making, the performing and the watching of them; and then includes them in a sequence of active processes of debate and reappraisal in which they can interrogate the systemic causes of the situations they face and decide on relevant action to be taken by the community in response.

DOI: 10.4324/9780429288753-1

The issues include provision of services (healthcare, education, electricity), functioning of local political and representative structures, rights, uses and abuses of land, response to state or central government policies, ingrained attitudes and practices (particularly patriarchy), specific threats to social and family life (illegal alcohol production, trafficking of women, girls, young people), and anything else which the communities they work in may face, including, most recently (2020), the effects of forced relocation of migrant workers from conurbations to the rural areas they originate from.

Sanjoy Ganguly, JS's artistic director, says that JS is an *activist movement*: theatre is a form and motivator of that activism, which is a mode of intervention by the people in the circumstances of their own lives and the structures which govern them. That movement centrally consists of a 'core team' of about 10–15 long-term practitioners, backed up by minimal administrative support, who function as actors, trainers, facilitators and local leaders in the communities from which most of them originated, and the 'satellite' teams and community organisational structures and ongoing activities which they have been instrumental in creating.

The principal members of the core team, in addition to Sanjoy Ganguly, are: Sima Ganguly, Satyaranjan Pal, Renuka Das, Pradeep Sardar, Pradeep Haldar, Pritilata Mondal, Kavita Bera, Chittaranjan Pramanik, Dipak Pal, Brindavan Halder, Rabin Jana, Sadananda Mondal, Jharna Mondal and Ambika Ganguly. Most of them split their time between the organisation's HQ and their own local areas. In addition to rehearsing and performing in Forum plays, they lead training, co-ordinate and direct local teams and are active in local social and political structures. Several of them function as Jokers for those teams.

Most JS plays are collectively scripted through workshops; the final script is crafted and directed by Sanjoy Ganguly. Local teams adjust scripts and initiate their own as necessary.

Sanjoy and Sima Ganguly come from Kolkata. Sanjoy gained a BA at Kolkata University and worked as a supervisor in an engineering firm before starting activist social and political work as a member of the Communist Party of India (Marxist). His father, initially an English teacher, took a job in accountancy to maintain his extended family, and was a respected community activist social worker and a Sanskrit scholar.

The other members of the core team are drawn from agricultural workers' families, from rural areas mainly to the south of Kolkata. Some of them began by working as day-labourers, hawkers and domestic workers.

In addition to the core team, there are around 30 local 'satellite' teams in the state of West Bengal, usually with about 12 members each, plus teams in neighbouring states – Jharkand, Tripura and Orissa. Since 1985 they have trained and developed around 50 teams. About half of the West Bengal teams are composed of women only (in a largely rural environment which is socially conservative and includes a large proportion of Muslim communities, this is significant).

In a typical year, Jana Sanskriti teams deliver approximately 100 performances every month to around 20,000 spectators, who are not charged admission. They estimate their activist base to be around 40,000.

Augusto Boal called JS the largest Theatre of the Oppressed movement in the world outside his native Brazil and afforded it a special status. JS has toured abroad several times; Ganguly has given many workshops throughout the world; many practitioners in India and beyond owe much of their training, perspective and methodology to him; as of 2020, JS has hosted seven biannual international festivals where practitioners and academics from all over the world have experienced its methods and its ambience; researchers are regularly to be found at JS's centre and work at all levels from BA dissertations to post-doctoral papers has explored its practice.

JS makes theatre in a particular way for particular purposes. It is more than a theatre company. For most of its 35-year life it has not primarily produced pre-scripted plays. It does not usually work in conventional theatres. It uses many processes which are recognisable to theatre students and practitioners, and draws on performance forms which derive from both local and international models, but has woven them into a style and a mode of operation which is specific to its context and its goals. These include key TO methodologies such as:

- *Image Theatre*: creating striking individual and collective physical images of conflict situations
- *theatre games and exercises*: developing expressive competence and confidence and leading to the production of scenarios which represent the participants' experience

- *Forum Theatre*: using a facilitator or 'Joker' to identify and open up key issues from the scenarios for debate through active participation. Spectators are invited to replace actors-in-role and rework key moments of the action; during these 'interventions', they become 'spect-actors'

Because of the kind of theatre they do and the way they do it, the movement extends to more than those who perform the plays.

> By Jana Sanskriti, I refer equally to the entire community of people – theatre teams in various villages, audiences, the central theatre team, urban, middle-class members – who have engaged in Jana Sanskriti's theatrical and political work and identify with central aspects of its political agenda. In this sense, Jana Sanskriti is a process rather than a bounded entity.
>
> (Mohan 2008: 4–5)

It is a theatre culture, a way of seeing and doing which touches many aspects of people's lives. Dia Da Costa (formerly Mohan), who has written about JS from a sociological and political perspective, calls it a 'process'; in addition, in terms of style, the theatre practice it operates is a distinctive mix of Boal's Theatre of the Oppressed and Indian folk culture, shaped by the specific contexts and challenges of a confrontational political landscape and a diverse population including Hindu, Muslim and tribal elements, with their own complex structures and relationships.

Some of the specifics may not be immediately accessible to people from other locations. Even Da Costa, who is Indian, says:

> I do not experience the daily violence of divisive party politics or the exploitation of market relations. Nor do I face extreme and consistent marginalization within processes of governance and citizenship. In short, I escape the most extreme forms of alienation in relations of production and representation.
>
> (Mohan 2008: 2)

As we will see, most of JS's members – actors, facilitators, community members – have faced and/or do face these kinds of situation regularly. However, if their situation is culturally, politically and historically specific, many elements of their work and its remit are both recognisable and transferable, and offer many possibilities of comparison, interrogation and challenge to practitioners and researchers across the world in the fields of Applied Theatre, Arts for Social Change and Theatre of the Oppressed, but also to those who have engaged with the relevance of theatre and arts practice to Development Studies, Communication Studies, Politics, Social Studies and other areas (see below and especially Chapters Two and Four).

This book explores all these aspects. It examines the contexts (geographical, historical, social, political and theatrical) in which JS works. It describes who comprises JS, what they do, how they do it and what the structures are which they have established to further this. It investigates what kinds of 'performance practice' this whole endeavour represents, what its significance is and what its outcomes and effects have been – in terms of productions, performances, ways of working, personal, social and community impact, and international connections. It also asks how much of this can be 'learned' by people who are not from India and who work in different places and contexts, and explores some of the ways that learning or transfer can take place.

The book has four chapters, which aim to articulate and situate JS's work and to make its practices accessible: Chapter One examines the history, contexts and goals of the work; Chapter Two interrogates key dimensions further with the help of what has been written about JS by its artistic director and others; Chapter Three looks closely at examples of its work in performance and as published scripts; and Chapter Four explores the kinds of exercises JS uses in training and play development.

In looking at these things, the book tries to articulate how the people who make up JS think, work, make theatre, understand its remit and view its impact. At every stage there are questions, direct or implied, about how and why, about the parameters and processes. The answers, by and large, are not simple, but they are the result of particular kinds of attitude and action. They offer possibilities of extending theatre processes and structures to engage with how people can understand, reflect (on) and negotiate their everyday contexts and the networks of influence which shape them. For JS, this means, as individuals and as part of communities and collectives, exploring the power of theatre to discover ways of speaking and acting in response to local and regional power structures (both political and religious), as means to influence the provision of services, and as kinds of behaviour which impact on how they live and work together.

For now, let's say JS is a way of making theatre, a network and practice of relationship, a developmental pedagogy and a structure of embodied politics.

LOCATION: BUILDING FROM THE GROUND UP

Jana Sanskriti is based in a rural location outside Kolkata, West Bengal. Established by Sanjoy Ganguly in 1985, it now has a training and administrative base at Girish Bhavan, Badu, named after Sri Girish Chandra Ghosh, a playwright, director, actor, lyricist and music composer in 19th century Bengal.

(Ganguly 2010: 1)

'Rural location' needs a little explanation. Badu, about 5km from the 'small' but very busy town of Madhyamgram and a little further from Barasat, is in a part of the North 24 Parganas district (north of Kolkata, not far from the airport) which is more like a kind of semi-rural ribbon development found extensively in India. Lots of narrow roads, houses and plots of various sizes, clusters (bazaars) of small informal shops, temples and mosques, rubbish, cows; masses of people, bicycles,

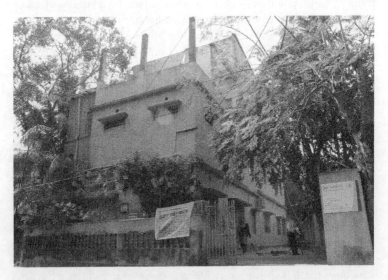

Figure 1.1 Girish Bhavan, Badu, Madhyamgram, Kolkata.

Photo: Jana Sanskriti

two-wheeled vehicles, auto-rickshaws, lorries, buses, noise, chaos; occasionally an emptyish space, a 'tank' or pond, maybe even a mango orchard, water-fowl, goats, chickens. Girish Bhavan was carved out of an overgrown bit of wilderness, the ground levelled, the building raised brick by brick, from a couple of office rooms and a verandah in the late 1990s to three floors, dormitory accommodation and a small theatre space in 2019 (the latter named the Augusto Boal auditorium and opened in 2015).

Food is cooked in the communal kitchen at the end of the plot, for all those who are there at any time: much of it organic, some grown in a plot next door, more (rice and dhal) in Digambapur, JS's base in the Ganges delta south of Kolkata. Making theatre goes hand in hand with building, growing crops, sharing all kinds of work. Activism takes many forms: it's a way of life, not a passing indulgence.

As Ganguly describes in his book, *Jana Sanskriti, Forum Theatre and Democracy in India* (2010), the impetus to using theatre came from his presence as an urban-educated political activist in a rural village. The section on company structures below and in Chapter Two of the book will explore this and other writing about JS in more detail and ask what key parameters about the work it articulates.

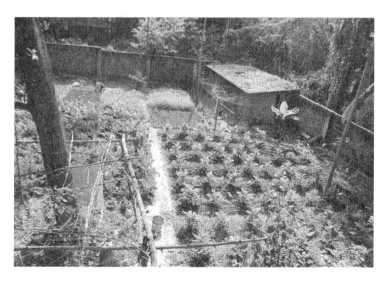

Figure 1.2 Kitchen garden, Badu.
Photo: Jana Sanskriti

So a little more about the history and geography is appropriate here, because it illustrates something about the ethos of the nascent entity which became Jana Sanskriti. The first phase runs from 1985 to 1997 and encompasses its initial work and the move to become an independent organisation. It started working in West Bengal villages in 1985; the core team was founded in 1986; Ganguly first came into contact with Boal's work in 1990–1.

In the early days in the small village of Milan More, to the south of Kolkata in the Ganges delta area known as the Sunderbans (much water, land regularly changing shape and form, mangrove swamps, but also extensive areas of good arable land with palms, rice paddy, ponds for fish, rice-straw-thatched villages among the trees), the team lived in a more or less derelict house by the side of a rural road. They were initially part of a larger social organisation, but began to develop the theatre work and discover their own identity in the process. Their first plays (*Gayer Panchali*, *Where We Stand*, *Shonar Meye*, *Sarama*) drew on central issues from the lives of the villagers and were created between 1987 and 1992. In 1991, Boal sent a team of French TO practitioners to run a workshop in West Bengal, and JS was invited to perform *Shonar Meye* in Paris.

In 1997, JS split from the West Bengal Agricultural Workers' Union and moved first to an even smaller location north of Kolkata in Barasat. By this time there were more members of the core team; they rehearsed, planned and often slept (up to 22 of them!) in the same room. Eventually they acquired some land in Badu. It was quite cheap, but Renuka Das says: 'it was like a jungle ... our members worked tirelessly to clear the space' (Das, in Da Costa 2010b: 52). When I conducted a workshop with them in 1999, in between sessions they would disappear: at first, I thought, for a siesta (they had been rehearsing with Ganguly before the workshop). But no, they were digging ditches, building walls. And then they came back to play theatre games!

What these brief images show is that they shared commitment, enthusiasm and a very basic life-style in which everyone contributed to the collective activity. That is still the pattern, if on a wider scale. So the structure has always been one of mutual support – several members tell stories about cycling miles to perform and walking together if one person got a puncture – and of contribution of what each person could offer, which was mostly practical skills, time and enthusiasm.

Later, the same kind of practical collaboration, coupled with some local donations, enabled JS to construct two rural performance spaces in the villages of Digambapur (1997) and Srinarayanpur (2010). These 'Mukta Mancha' serve also as meeting places and venues for many kinds of cultural, educational, social and political events for the village throughout the year. They also consciously signal JS's conviction that 'culture' is directly related to and fundamentally supportive of everyday life and that it is for everyone, not just the urban or 'intellectual' elite.

Jana Sanskriti was initially part of another social movement, West Bengal Agricultural Workers' Union. In his book *Forum Theatre and Democracy in India*, Sanjoy Ganguly tells the story of leaving the Communist Party, working in the slums in Kolkata, meeting migrant labourers from rural districts and going to their villages to experience their situation at first hand (Ganguly 2010: 8). He was already uneasy with the way that cultural practice was relegated to the status of a support service in the CPM (Communist Party of India: Marxist); it often served to attempt to persuade the audience that the Party had their interests at heart and to explain and promote its policies. This sense of impotence was compounded by the situation within the social movement, where JS was regarded as something like a 'cultural wing'. In reality, it was doing most of the grass-roots interactive work, engaging with the people and beginning to listen rather than attempt to persuade. From 1991, JS became increasingly uneasy with this position, and this eventually (in 1997) led to a split on ethical and ideological grounds.

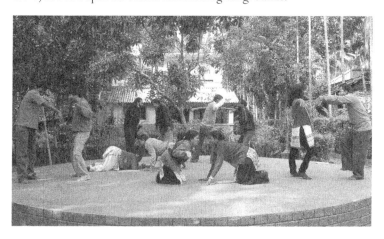

Figure 1.3 Outside stage at Girish Bhavan.

Photo: Jana Sanskriti

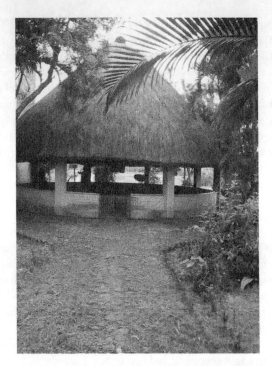

Figure 1.4 The Mukta Manch at Digambapur, S. 24 Parganas, West Bengal.

Photo: Ralph Yarrow

Prior to 1992, the theatre work followed a more 'top-down' format, along the lines of message-delivery through art operated by political parties, NGOs or urban intellectual well-wishers (rather like 'agit-prop' in Soviet Russia, early 'Theatre for Development' in Africa), because that was what Ganguly was familiar with. However, several key insights (see Chapters Two and Three) led him and the small group who stuck it out in the villages with him to begin to work in a different way, which exemplified many of the characteristics of TO, although he did not at first have any knowledge of that. The first contact with Boal arose within the combined unit; the visit of a team of trainers sent by Boal from CTO/Cétidade Paris – Jean-François Martel and four others – followed by JS's own trip to Paris in 1991, fell within this period, and the reception JS received there strengthened their self-belief. Ganguly read parts of Boal's *Theatre of the Oppressed* during this time, and became aware that Boal's model of a socially embedded form of theatre, which did not 'talk down' to its audience or impose one point of view, was what JS was already in large measure beginning to do. In Paris they also met Boal in person; he was hugely impressed by the aesthetic and dramaturgical qualities of their play *Shonar Meye* (*Golden Girl*), about stages of a woman's life, and formed a strong bond with Ganguly. From 1997, JS became an independent organisation, in part assisted by Ganguly's receipt of a Fellowship from the Indian office of the Macarthur Foundation. (Macarthur India grants supported work in education, human rights and the environment. Ganguly's was one of eight awards in 1997.) Though the award was not on the scale of the Fellowships awarded in the USA, Ganguly felt unable to accept the lump sum involved and requested that he should receive only the salary component, which enabled the group to look for its own headquarters and was used for the land purchase. In response, the Foundation extended the salary for a further two years, which helped to establish JS's independent existence.

JS had already co-operated with other activist and socially engaged groups across India on a 55-day bicycle rally to Delhi, in support of a basic work-guarantee for agricultural workers in 1989 (doing performances each evening as they went); subsequently JS reached out to many other such groups to introduce them to TO methodology, and Ganguly delivered workshops across the country. Funding from these – and subsequently from workshops abroad – was ploughed back into the company; the contacts also led to the foundation of the Indian Federation of the Theatre of the Oppressed (FOTO), inaugurated in person by Augusto Boal in 2006. In a sense, JS is thus born from this division, this fundamental *prise de position*, which clarifies its status and underlying beliefs and begins to lay the foundation for a distinctive working practice. Above all, this can be summed up in the distinction between theatre *for* the oppressed and theatre *of* the oppressed, which remains the key plank of Ganguly's and JS's position.

The dates in the box chart the developing strands of JS's work: training, development of dramaturgies and plays, community activism and organisation, international connectivities. The following sections explore these and other dimensions in detail, and begin to explain how they interrelate and emerge in parallel as JS learned from its experiences.

Important dates

1985 Beginnings in West Bengal villages; first teams formed

1986 Core team founded

1990/1 Ganguly first reads short sections of Boal's work

1991 Boal sends team of French TO practitioners to run workshop in West Bengal
JS perform *Shonar Meye* in Paris

1987–92 First plays: *Gayer Panchali*, *Where We Stand*, *Shonar Meye*,
Sarama

1992 Boal sends Ganguly *Games for Actors and Non-Actors*

1994 Boal gives workshop in India

1995 First cycle rally to Delhi

1997 JS split from West Bengal Agricultural Workers' Union;
MacArthur award; move to Barasat, then Badu: Girish Bhavan
phase 1 constructed; Mukta Manch constructed in Digambapur

1997/8 JS participate in Seagull workshop, Kolkata

2002 Village committees start; first all-women teams

2004 First Muktadhara International Festival of Forum Theatre
(biannual> 2018)

2006 Major rally in Kolkata with Augusto Boal; Indian Federation
of TO established

2008 JS participate in protests against car factory in Singhur,
West Bengal

2011–15 First 'foreign' play by JS: *The Village Dream*

2015 JSIRRI (Jana Sanskriti International Research and Resource
Institute) inaugurated
Augusto Boal auditorium opened at Girish Bhavan

2018 Ganguly awarded Ibsen Fellowship; *A Doll's House* (*Khelar Ghor*)

2019 Jana Sanskriti Diploma in Applied Theatre launched

THEATRE OF THE OPPRESSED AND
FORUM THEATRE

Jana Sanskriti makes Forum Theatre. Beyond this, the *methodology of Forum* characterises its practice in many dimensions. This means that shared input and a critical attitude underpin the work.

Jana Sanskriti's practice is to compose scenes and shape them into plays during workshops with the community, drawing on their experience of issues which affect them. They then use a mix of **Image Theatre** (which employs the resources of the body, individually or collectively, to create readable signs of social situations) and **folk music, folk dance and folk theatre styles** to help script and present them. Initially the largely co-created script emerges as a sequence of images, to which words and actions are added in stages (see Chapter Four for detailed examples of how this works by using sets of games and exercises). What emerges is a particular model of **Forum Theatre**.

The **Forum Theatre** process invites audience members firstly to reflect on the performance they have seen, to evaluate how accurate it is as a representation of their reality, to decide how they feel about the outcome and, then, crucially, to begin to analyse the underlying structural causes of the oppression (social, interpersonal, economic, political, etc.). This initial interactive section is facilitated by a 'Joker' who engages the audience and encourages responses and discussion, and then invites them to become 'spect-actors': to come on stage, embody and act out as well as verbalise alternative choices at key moments in the action. But the remaining actors, who play roles of other interested parties – who may represent various kinds of vested interests or simply 'bystanders' – resist any simple revision or 'magic solution', and stick to their entrenched or exploitative positions, so that a conflict is engendered. Each 'intervention' is pursued and problematised as far as possible; and then, at a point where it is clear what it has to offer, is suspended by the Joker, in order to allow further proposals to be explored. In this way, a series of more or less plausible responses to the original situation are played out and, implicitly and explicitly, compose a kind of dialogue to which the spectators and spect-actors contribute on equal terms with the original actors. A concluding discussion assesses the relative merits of the proposed interventions, pointing 'beyond the stage' to possible courses of political action.

In Forum, the play or scenes from it are performed and examined several times. The first run of all the scenes usually lasts between 20 and 30 minutes. Subsequent discussion and interaction often extends far longer – in the case of Jana Sanskriti normally for two hours or more.

Frances Babbage writes that the aim of Forum 'is twofold: to find ways to combat a specific oppression, and to create maximum opportunity for participation' (Babbage 2004: 142). Dia Mohan/Da Costa exemplifies this in JS's practice as a way of debating the social context of a problem such as domestic violence through engaging in scripting plays (Mohan 2008: 5); Sameera Iyengar notes that Forum discourages simplistic solutions in favour of thorough analysis (Iyengar 2001: 90). The Forum experience functions rather like a 'change-lab', an intensive experimental situation which Adam Kahane describes as follows:

a controlled environment within which a group of people experience, become conscious of, and then develop strategies to cope with the turbulent and fast-moving dynamic of a modern society. In comparison with the 'real' world, the change lab aspires to be a space within which it is safe to do things differently, be that shifting power relations or fostering a culture where mistakes are the basis of learning.

(Kahane 2010: 122–3)

This closely resembles Boal's and JS's descriptions of the Forum process as a 'safe space' within which potential shifts of power, relations, attitudes and behaviours can occur in the form of 'rehearsals for reality'.

In this intensive and extensive process, both bodies and intellects are activated; the theatre space becomes an arena for dialogue, a mirror, a space for reflection and collective research, which draws on the capacities of all present. Thus, in TO, the audience ceases to be merely receptive – or, as Boal claims in respect of 'classical' theatre, passive – and becomes active: as 'spect-actors' they explore, show, analyse and transform the reality in which they are living: initially conceptually, but then in increasing ways as practice, beginning with 'acting it out' on stage, which Boal sees as a 'rehearsal for revolution'; then taking it into 'joint social action' (Ganguly 2010: 88–9; 137) (reflecting on, contributing to an understanding of the dimensions of the situation) and further into individual or communal direct activist engagement (protests, marches, deputations to local government offices, intervention in local political forums, establishment of proactive groups, etc.).

Forum methodology here materialises Boal's political, educational and developmental aims, articulated in the *Declaration of Principles of Theatre of the Oppressed* (reproduced in Fritz 2016: 69ff; 293–5).

The title of Boal's pivotal work, *Theatre of the Oppressed*, derives from the 'pedagogy of the oppressed' articulated by his friend and Brazilian compatriot Paulo Freire. Freire's book (1970) argues for the recognition and validation of practical, embodied and multi-generic skills and knowledges on a par with the verbal and exclusively intellectual, and for a model of learning as exchange between equals.

Ganguly sees Boal's desire 'to humanise humanity' by recognising the intelligence of everyone, as an essential first step in returning to the people the power to create, which enables them to recognise and deploy their status (a slight amendment of Karl Marx's idea of returning the means of production to the people), thereby valuing their labour and empowering them to 'own' the resources which they possess and deploy.

So from this perspective, TO is not just making productions about social and political realities, although that is at its heart. Identifying, analysing and evaluating that reality, whilst collaboratively crafting the production and further interrogating and critiquing it during the performance, activates intellectual and creative agency and allows participants to engage in renegotiating the parameters of their lives. Issues like the dowry system, the use and ownership of land and the provision of education are fundamental to those lives (others are mentioned below and in the account of plays in Chapter Three); they are workshopped, crafted into plays and performed by and for those whom they affect.

POLITICAL CONTEXT

In JS's play *Sarama*, a character comments: 'So this state power is for the Party, not for people. The Party is not there to serve people. The people are there to serve the Party' (*Sarama*, in Ganguly 2009: 86). Precisely for this reason, JS adopted a form of practice which would offer the possibility of challenging political hierarchy and assumptions of power and intellectual prestige by a form of theatre which makes clear that the people possess the intellectual and organisational capacity to address the issues which impact on their lives themselves. However, at the heart of the process of Forum is the awareness that challenge by itself is not enough.

When Jana Sanskriti was founded in 1985, West Bengal was governed by a Left Front Government (LFG) from 1977 to 2011, with the Communist Party of India (Marxist) (CPM) at its head. This government achieved considerable land reform and economic redistribution via the *panchayat* (village governance) system, but as time went on, it shifted its agenda 'from radical transformation to the mechanisms through which to deliver development and ensure electoral stability' (Mohan 2008: 3) – which included negotiating with industrialists (notably the huge Indian/multinational conglomerate Tata) who wanted to acquire agricultural land in order to build manufacturing plant. Relatively soon, it became clear that the CPM was more interested in the appearance of democracy than the reality. Mohan points out that 'while the CPM has given marginalized … people *access* to representation … the party has ensured that people never come to *control* the terms and the meaning of representation and their participation in these processes' (2008: 3; emphasis in original): in other words, the local representatives didn't have a say in who was in charge of the agenda and how decisions were taken.

Thus the model of theatre operated by JS was specifically developed to shift the dynamics of this situation and make a genuine addition to local democracy. Over the course of its existence, JS has never accepted funding from political parties; but it has nevertheless had to recognise and negotiate with local structures emanating from those parties, through which the provision of services is often channelled: a delicate and often difficult balancing act, complicated by the fact that during its period in government the CPM was opposed, and from 2011 replaced in power, by the Trinamul Congress. Conflict between these parties has frequently been violent and both have attempted to control areas and dominate local power hierarchies.

Jana Sanskriti has developed theatre teams in various villages in West Bengal and in other regions of India. Each of these theatre teams combines activity onstage with activism offstage within the villages in which the theatre teams are formed. Dia Mohan writes:

> [t]here are two integral **practices** to Jana Sanskriti's work: performances and fieldwork. The first practice involves rehearsals, theatre workshops, enactment of plays, engagement in Forum Theatre, and organizing cultural festivals. The second involved the process of calling meetings, discussion and debate groups, brainstorming sessions, 'ideological training'.
>
> (Mohan 2008: 4)

The teams join with members of the community to:

> engage in bargaining with the **panchayat** for the right to cultural spaces, fighting dowry and domestic violence, mobilizing people to participate in cultural activities, demanding the right to work in the villages rather than being dependent on migration for work, and mobilizing anti-liquor agitations.
>
> (Mohan 2008: 4)

The North and South 24 Parganas districts (north and south of Kolkata) have been major centres of JS activity (the districts are divided into administrative 'blocks', and JS has had strong presence in particular in two blocks in S24 Parganas – Kulpi and Pathar Pratima); more recently they have also developed teams in Purulia (north-west of Kolkata). Many parts of these districts are characterised by relatively poor or imbalanced service provision (e.g. of roads, electricity, access to healthcare facilities, primary education). The region also has a high proportion of Muslim inhabitants and provision sometimes reflects both this and differences in caste. Approximately 30–33% of JS's spectator community is Muslim (Ganguly 2010: 124). In the areas in which JS work, there is also a similar proportion of Dalit ('Scheduled Caste'/' Scheduled Tribe') population.

West Bengal has over 97 million inhabitants (2018 figure); Jana Sanskriti estimate that in a year, approximately 200,000 people have – often quite extensive and prolonged – exposure to their work.

Indian political structures

National Government (Delhi): **National Assembly**

currently Bharatiya Janata Party (BJP) (right wing); previously, Congress Party (centre left) held power for 54 years between 1947 (Independence) and 2014

State Governments (**Local Assemblies**) in 28 states (+ 8 Union Territories)

In West Bengal, currently Trinamul Congress (TRC); previously, Communist Party of India (Marxist) (CPM) in power as part of Left Front Government (LFG) from 1977–2011

Local administration is organised via Districts, Blocks and the *gram panchayat* (village level) system

West Bengal has 10 Districts, including Kolkata, North and South 24 Parganas

There are 29 Blocks in S24 Parganas including Pathar Pratima and Kakdwip

There are 310 *gram panchayat* in S24 Parganas

The areas in which JS operate have thus been marked by strong Party political activity and power struggles in which both (now, since the BJP is also making considerable gains, three) Party groupings are similarly authoritarian and aggressive. Parties adopt issues and claim to speak for sections of the population in order to attract voters, which has continuously led to violent confrontations. JS members' and spectator communities' lives have been directly impacted by many of the issues mentioned above, and by others like corruption in the police and in government, which has occurred under both regimes. Since JS explicitly foregrounds both the issues and the political infighting which surrounds them, impartially exposing those from all sides who engage in it, they have not infrequently been attacked by all Parties. Ganguly reports one such incident in Midnapore in 1991. Following a production of JS's play *Where We Stand*, which questions political violence, the team were 'in a meeting with some spectators', when they were attacked by a mob who 'destroyed some mud walls to get in and beat us'. Ganguly was 'forced to go to a club house', where the leaders insisted that he should eat some rice. Suspecting that it was poisoned, he refused, but even when he was released had to leave the village by an alternative route in order to avoid another attack (Ganguly 2010: 80).

Dia Mohan suggests that JS's theatre practice is an effective and legitimate form of political action, for the following reasons:

- they have built a community of people who come together to express their critique and construction of social relations and alternate futures onstage
- they offer a significant space for people to express alternate visions of relations with urban markets, political systems and service provision, as well as with local politicians, patriarchs, development practitioners and landowners
- they provide the chance to build 'relations of cooperation rather than relations of competition and division historically nourished by party political rule and market relations'
- they open the possibility of 'learn[ing] how to and teach[ing] others how to commit themselves to living new commitment offstage' (Mohan 2008: 7)

REACHING OUT: COMMITTEES AND COMMUNITY STRUCTURES; SOCIAL AND PARTICIPATORY PRACTICES AIMED AT CASCADING/MULTIPLYING AND DEVELOPING SUSTAINABILITY

At the same time that they were establishing the Badu base (from 1997), JS was also developing its reach into rural communities, initially to the south of Kolkata and later both towards the north-west and beyond the state boundaries. This horizontal development aimed to extend the impact of the work both geographically and structurally; it was guided by insights derived from experience and by a clear understanding of the essential principles of participatory action which are themselves embedded in the methodology of Forum practice. The goal was to cascade the qualities of theatrical and social practice as JS understood and operated them as profoundly as possible, so that communities could create their own autonomous teams of actor-activists which would be supported by relevant and effective structures. As this endeavour progressed it traced out more and more ways in which a practice based in relationship and collaboration could begin to shift social and political norms.

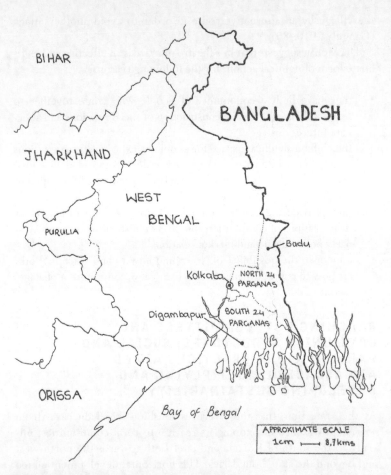

Figure 1.5 JS's operational areas in West Bengal.

Credit: Zorya Yarrow

Da Costa (2010a) identifies three channels along which JS interacts with a community:

- the establishment and organisation of committees and local political or semi-political structures
- involvement with service provision or issues (e.g. engagement in educational institutions or participation in actions to impact conditions)
- delivery of public events (i.e. theatre work)

All of these require extensive groundwork in order to integrate them into local structures and behaviours. These channels developed simultaneously because JS started not by 'parachuting in' with ready-made solutions to what they thought might be the issues to address, but by embedding themselves within the localities and discovering as they went along, in conjunction with the local inhabitants, what kinds of methodology and what kinds of support structures were most effective.

The first dimension of this multi-layered strategy is repetition of the performance itself:

> In a process of alternation, which encourages experience, reflection and analysis, the forum event is repeated at least three times at short intervals (1–3 months) for the same audience (in a village or rural centre). The forum process allows the issue to be opened up for discussion and comment and encourages 'interventions' which suggest strategies to address it. On subsequent occasions, the same spectators engage repeatedly with the issue in order to be able to do so from increasing degrees of understanding and with increasingly sophisticated and imaginative levels of response.

(Yarrow 2017: 30)

The sequences of engagement JS use – which include but are not limited to Performance > Forum > Intervention> Workshop > Rehearsal – function as a process of mutuality and exchange. Performances, as noted above, are repeated at least three times to the same audience. Audiences are encouraged (by the Joker during the performance but also by other members of the performance team in the run-up to performance and in the intervals between performances) to reflect upon and analyse the structural causes of the incidents and issues depicted, in a 'Brechtian' manner: not to accept them passively or be seduced by their spectacular nature, but to question them. At the same time, they are invited to be physically as well as mentally active, to intervene in the repeated version of a scene or situation and to articulate a verbal or physical response.

'Repetition is a powerful tool in this theatre because it gives people the time and space to nurture their confidence' (and also to 'try again' if proposed solutions on- or offstage 'reach dead-ends') (Mohan 2008: 6). The community, therefore, is gradually enabled to explore as many of the resonances and dissonances of issues which affect them as possible, and given the means to contribute to the 'rehearsal' and application of strategies to address them; the tenor of the experience, its physical texture as it were within the communal as well as individual body, is altered. 'Theatre' here becomes an ongoing life event and strategy, delivered in and by the participating bodies, individual and collective. The repetition over a period of time also recognises that 'issues' take time and tenacity to resolve; as proposed remedies are debated and tried out, the shape of the problem may alter, new strategies may be called for: the community is being 'trained' to think on its feet and respond imaginatively, astutely and courageously in a process of ongoing improvisation, delivery, assessment, re-evaluation and reconfiguration: acting is gradually but profoundly transformed into activism, spect-actors – as Ganguly has delightedly and appropriately extemporised – into 'spect-activists' (Ganguly 2017: 136).

The kinds of issues addressed have been outlined above and will also be identified via the examination of JS's plays in Chapter Three. They are also referred to by JS core team members writing in Da Costa's edited collection of essays about JS, *Scripting Power*: Renuka Das describes an anti-liquor agitation; she and Pradeep Haldar speak of action to improve education facilities; Pradeep Sardar describes working on the play about people living below the poverty line (Da Costa 2010b: 54–6, 65, 81–2). From these and other accounts, it is clear that although each issue or point of focus has its own temporal and political identity, they frequently run into or affect each other and are all linked by many threads of influence, behaviour, conditions of life and so on. The anti-liquor action was led by women, coming together and acting in defiance of the police and the suppliers; more recent work to counteract trafficking has united communities and redefined responsibilities. JS's careful integration into this web of events and processes is vital to the instigation of these far-reaching social and political changes.

The same is true of the ways in which local residents engage with the work. Some audience members may become 'spect-actors' in Forum events; all of them will at least be present and be invited to participate in the alternation of experience and reflection, which the Forum sets in motion. Others will be affected more indirectly by discussion of those events and by shifts in behaviour or attitude within their often close-knit community. To whatever degree the participants subsequently engage in discussion within their community, they enter a further level of activation, which is supported by the establishment, in many areas of West Bengal in which Jana Sanskriti works, of committees, which began in

2002 and has increased over the years. Originally called 'spect-actors' committees', they are now known as Human Rights Protection Committees and Responsible Citizens' Committees, in recognition of their status, remit and agency. In a further extension, many locations in which JS works have now also instituted 'watch committees' (e.g. keeping an eye on any attempts to traffic women and young people) and 'mothers' forums' (which discuss issues related to education, children and women in general). These groups have arisen from engagement with problems and issues which have featured in plays and resultant action. Their task is to identify issues which can form the subject of future performances and community action, organise these events and keep people talking about the issues. In most cases, the members of these committees are themselves either performers who have followed the training process or fairly regular spect-actors who offer interventions at Forum events. So here both 'practice' and 'performance' acquire extended meaning: they are forms of action which impact many strata of community behaviour, as a number of wide-ranging studies have confirmed (see e.g. Hoff et al. 2021, discussed further in Chapter Two).

The performances also serve to recruit new performers, often from among women and young people. These people then undergo training provided through workshops by the existing local 'satellite team', if there is one, and/or by members of the core team. They thus embark on a relatively recognisable trajectory from trainee/participant/performer to trainer/artistic leader (see also Chapter Four). This trajectory involves the acquisition of skills and techniques, ways of drawing on performance knowledges, techniques of developing co-creativity and collaborative scripting and the extension of these capacities to community activism. So it locates resources in the minds and bodies of individuals, moulds and hones them through practice, nourishes and deepens them through interaction, continued debate and experimentation, and deploys and tests them against real-life challenges in the social and political world. JS's work thus leads to 'direct action well beyond the theatre space' through 'genuinely collective processes that generate critical thinking that is never finished' (Eugene van Erven in Ganguly 2017: xii).

This ongoing developmental process has evolved in response to a situation in which the concept of 'the people' tends to be constructed – by political parties and the instruments of government which they oversee or influence – as a passive and manipulable entity. JS's shift away from a similarly 'top-down' mode of theatre is one of its early key realisations. Both in the encounter of Forum, built around critique and 'rational collective action', on and offstage, and in the formation and operation of committees and community engagement groups, JS's audiences and participant groups defy norms; they 'refuse to play normative scripts loyally' (Da Costa 2010b: 626) – where the words 'play' and 'scripts' relate to both on- and offstage activity. Theatre is not just entertainment or diversion, but also a challenge to who you are and how you act; knowing your place is what you assume responsibility for, not what you take 'for granted'.

Liberal-capitalist models of 'development' largely frame it in economic terms which overlook the human value of the workers who deliver it. The CPM/LFG, although avowedly at the other end of the political spectrum, in practice operated a similar attitude of top-down hegemony towards actual people. For Ganguly, JS's work is 'development [in a very different sense] because it [fights] the violence and divisive effects of all forms of instrumentalist politics on human relationship' (Mohan 2008: 3). Whereas these negate or marginalise the inherent capacities of the very people they claim to assist, JS uses the interpersonal processes of theatre to realise them more fully.

If, for JS, 'theatre is not enough', neither is politics, which, like capitalism, has tended to 'instrumentalise' human capacity instead of nourishing it. So JS's understanding and deployment of the relationship factors embedded in theatre process is a psychosocial, autopoietic and ethical aesthetic. It also interprets the concept of 'political action' in a more complex way. Because they work in and with communities, they recognise the 'complexities of social inequalities' and other factors, register the nuances of interaction between factions, families, hierarchies and strata, and, instead of simply prescribing a 'programme', use the interactive and communicative qualities of seeing, questioning and commenting on, and making theatre together as an ongoing pedagogy for change. The notion of 'community' itself is of course problematic; it may conceal assumptions about homogeneity, or run risks of nostalgia for an imagined past or ideal. JS's embedding in the locations where they perform means that they recognise this and work with it. Their Forum and committee operation targets 'a rainbow of differing opinions, rather than a consensual homogeneity of opinion' (Neelands in Prendergast and Saxton 2009: 29).

In the villages where JS has worked over a period of time, people see and meet each other differently, behave in different ways towards each other, as spectators and possibly spect-actors, as participants in sessions to 'script' their own realities, as players in training games and in the interrogative and combative 'game' of Forum Theatre. One area in which this is particularly evident is the increasing participation of women: at the beginning, most of the performers were men; gradually, 'wives and daughters' began to join, and in so doing to acquire increasing status and confidence, until in some cases all-women teams were formed, beginning in 2002 (core team members Priti Mondal and Pradeep Sardar write about this also in Da Costa 2010b: 66, 71–2) and the gender make-up of the organisation moved towards its current situation, in which women have at least equal presence in terms of performers, leadership roles and active engagement. Thus 'Jana Sanskriti seemed to people to be a part of their landscape' (Da Costa 2008: 10), as opposed to the irregular visits of entertainment or educational performances. They are continually referred to as living evidence of a 'culture' which is rooted in the everyday experience of the inhabitants. Even more, over the years JS team members have come to be recognised, sometimes formally but also informally, as channels of assistance and advice in many respects. Whether or not the particular need is taken up in a play or in community action, JS provides an avenue for beginning to address it – locating doctors, giving assistance with writing letters, raising issues in village or local forums and so on.

So JS's version of what in TO circles (e.g. at CTO Rio) is often referred to as 'multiplying' is very broadly based; it 'cascades' processes, practices and structures into the environment and thus underpins deep social transformation. Although individual performances and campaigns are very important, they are the point of an arrow: ongoing presence and a repertoire of modes of engagement mean that change is occurring at the level of community beliefs, behaviours and relationships. These are reflected in long-term shifts in social practice reported by members over the years (e.g. ceasing to ask for dowry; extending support for girls' education) and reported in essays by the core team (in Da Costa 2010b); evaluative studies of behavioural shifts indicate similar parameters (Hoff et al. 2021 and Brahma et al. 2019).

In a further sense of environment, JS's work also redefines both performance space and public space (see discussion of Clément Poutot's work in Chapter Two); the former in the Boalian sense of reducing the

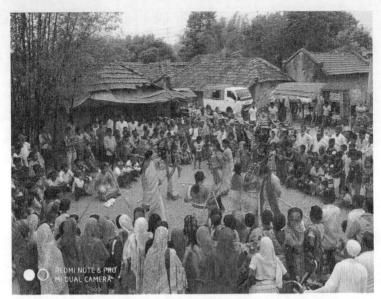

Figure 1.6 JS performance in Tetulia village, Pathar Pratima block, South 24
        Parganas (a strongly Muslim area).

Photo: Jana Sanskriti

Author's note: in 2016, I saw a new team of young JS performers do the first play in a similar
village. At the meeting of four ways. Adjacent to a temple on one side and a mosque on
the other, evidence of the meeting of beliefs and people. They came and watched. They
understood and reflected, shouted out responses and suggestions. One by one they came
into the space of the action and took part, proposed other versions of the narrative. At the
back of the audience, a noisy group debated excitedly. They said: 'You must come again.
This is the first time we've been asked what we think.'

distinction between stage and audience in terms of agency and physicality, in that they normally perform on the same level as and often
surrounded closely by the audience; the latter in the way they '[offer] a
significant space for people to express their alternate visions of relations
with urban markets, political systems, and health centers as well as with
local politicians, patriarchs, development practitioners and landowners'
(Da Costa 2008: 7). In doing this and doing it in 'found' or 'converted'
spaces (often a courtyard, school, field or street), 'everyday arenas of
Bengal's rural landscape [are] legitimized as new space for governance'
(ibid: 7).

INTERNAL DEMOCRACY

In its function as a movement, JS has a number of levels of accountability and planning. They include the committees referred to in the foregoing sections, plus a General Council and an Executive Committee. (FOTO, The Indian Federation of Theatre of the Oppressed, has its own committee.) JS is registered as a Society under Indian law and has to fulfil all tax requirements accordingly (it's not an NGO).

JS structures

Core team (10–15; shifts between Badu HQ and villages)
    30+ satellite teams (8–12 in each; mainly in W. Bengal, others in Orissa, Tripura, Jharkand etc.)
    General Council (60 members) drawn from all teams: formulates policy, agrees initiatives
    Human Rights Protection Committees (HRPCs), Watch Committees, Mothers' Forums
    (village and district level: promote and oversee actions, organise performances etc.)
    links with teams/movements in Delhi, Maharashtra etc.
    JS teams deliver approx. 100 performances per year to 200,000 spectators
    Plays and actions address
    provision of services (healthcare, education, electricity)
    functioning of local political and representative structures
    rights, uses and abuses of land
    responses to State or Central government policies
    ingrained attitudes and practices (particularly patriarchy)
    specific threats to social and family life: illegal alcohol production, trafficking of women, girls, young people

---

'The General Council is composed of members from each satellite team and takes all important decisions, while the Executive Committee [a legal entity required by Indian law] implements the decisions taken by General Council' (Sima Ganguly, in Da Costa 2010b: 44). In effect this means all full-time JS workers and at least one representative from each team form the General Council of 60 members, which meets four times a year and discusses all planning, projects and organisational matters.

These committees operate what Sanjoy Ganguly calls 'consensus politics', which means essentially that they work by collective agreement rather than by numerical voting. In particular the General Council meets not for a few hours but over two (usually very long) days, so that there is time to discuss extensively, allow time for reflection and arrive at a consensus.

As already noted, Jana Sanskriti is more than a circumscribed entity. It's a process, a network and an extended set of interactions within communities. So it's more than a company in the usual sense of the word. Of course all theatre companies are complemented by, justified by, supported by the publics they engage with. But in most cases these elements are fluid, in the sense that the individuals who compose them change over time, and are linked to the company by interest – which may vary from production to production – rather than by necessity or direct relevance to the contexts and conditions of their everyday lives. In JS's case, the community *is* their work. The aim is not just entertainment or even just intellectual or aesthetic stimulation, but rather a combination of all these in an evaluation of and encounter with the fundamentals of the lived circumstances which issues as action.

So its structures are more extensive, in dimension and in kind. Within the core group of performers and senior trainers itself, decisions (about issues to address, plays to create or re-perform, new groups to develop, etc.) are taken collectively, after extensive debate and without a vote. The latter is important. Until everyone agrees, that step is not taken.

In his 2010 book *Jana Sanskriti: Forum Theatre and Democracy in India*, Ganguly recounts a kind of parable: a man is found to have been stealing and the village leaders discuss his punishment. Everyone except one person agrees that he should pay a fine. They think some more, and then one of them says: 'it's like the nets we use for fishing; they're held apart by sticks. If one stick falls out, you can still use the net. But sooner or later, the whole thing will fall apart.' They agree not to make him pay the fine (Ganguly 2010: n.6 to Ch. 9, 157–8).

There's an understanding and a principle at work here which says a lot about the way JS views community: not only views it, but constructs it. Democracy is more than just having a vote (although that is important). It's about thinking beyond immediate outcomes to the structures which underpin relationships and practices, and about sometimes doing what may seem illogical or contradictory, not simply trying for a quick consensus. That's how they do life as well as plays.

FUNDING AND FINANCE

JS receives no money from State or national government and does not accept funding from political parties. Most of its funding is short term and linked to specific projects consistent with its goals and practices. Recently its work in Purulia has been supported by the Commonwealth Foundation, and work in Pathar Pratima block of South 24 Parganas is supported by a grant from the Paul Hamlyn Foundation. Previously work has been funded by grants from the Prince Claus Fund and the Tata Trust. Da Costa (2010a: 628) notes that earlier funding for work in schools came from ICICI Bank and Tata. At early stages of its independent existence it received some money from the Sangeet Natak [Performing Arts] Academy, and a salary grant from the Macarthur Foundation. Other income to support satellite teams and ongoing work is derived from giving workshops in India and abroad and occasional teaching by Ganguly in universities, from performances abroad by the core team and from donations. HRPCs are financially autonomous and raise the funds they need to fulfil their function.

JS's ethics mean that it does not accept commissions from funders or intermediaries (e.g. NGOs) which do not match its principles. As a result its salary scale is far lower than that offered by many other groups. JS has a minimal office staff and has not been able to employ professional fundraisers. When money runs short (e.g. between grants), all members vote on how to deal with the situation – which may not infrequently mean that they agree to a cut in salary.

Birgit Fritz however makes an important observation about this state of affairs:

> The practice of TO as JS is living it is not about projects with deadlines and funding that can run out any time. It is an informed and felt decision, a determination to live and to dream life differently than the mainstream culture of monologue wants us to believe is possible …
>
> (Fritz 2016: 171)

Funding is indeed both tenuous and necessary. But for JS, the desire to do the work is bigger than the funding. I have heard Sanjoy and Sima

Ganguly, Satyaranjan Pal and others say often that they operate on the principle that if they believe the work is vital, they do it and trust that the money will turn up at some point. From a 'realistic' point of view that looks like impossible idealism. Sanjoy also often makes the perhaps surprising point that it is an entirely pragmatic necessity to 'romanticise optimism'; in other words, you need a vision to keep you going, whilst remaining quite clear that it is a long-term goal and that its stages need continuous critique. And as we have seen, JS has already kept going, somewhat impossibly, for more than 30 years. Maybe this is another dimension in which their practice challenges received wisdom. It is certainly part of the way in which they combine dimensions of operation which most contemporary attitudes would find difficult or embarrassing to run together. Economics and love? Nonsense, of course. Committees and consensus? Quite impractical. JS does both. And against a background fraught with multiple material hurdles.

THE THEATRE CONTEXT: ASPECTS OF THE POST-INDEPENDENCE INDIAN THEATRE SCENE

After Independence (1947), Indian theatre reflected the crucial need to formulate a 'national identity'. Not surprisingly, this has been complex and contentious. On the one hand it meant engaging in debates about *form*: what kinds of performance form are specifically Indian, how can they be accessed and their distinctiveness marked and asserted? It also involved issues of *content*, relating to Indian history and to the vision of a new country – again, unsurprisingly, complex and contentious. This of course is a very wide-angle vision. It's here in order to signal that some of the things that distinguish JS's performance – issues and aesthetics central amongst them – were the subject of intense debate over many decades across India. A useful way of getting a sense of this in more detail is to dip into *Seagull Theatre Quarterly* (*STQ*), a journal published from Kolkata between 1994 and 2003 (accessible at http://www.seagullindia.com/wordpress1/seagull-theatre-quarterly/) which has interviews with writers, directors and performers, and discussions of plays and events. A major topic is the recourse to 'folk' and 'tradition', by largely urban, middle-class artists ('Theatre of Roots') which, although producing some lively and often politically astute theatre, could also be charged with suggesting a kind of mythological Indianness which ignored the multiple differences of class, caste, culture, language and economic distinction which exist in such a vast country.

Both form and content are linked to politics in a variety of senses. The following snapshot doesn't cover all the angles and overlaps, but aims to sketch out the main parameters.

Between 1947 and roughly 1980, work mainly falls into three major formal strands: 'Street theatre', 'Theatre of Roots' and social realism.

- *Street theatre*: short message-oriented plays addressing economic and political issues (workers' rights etc.); performed in public spaces (factory yards, street corners); an alternative to the colonialist model of the proscenium-arch 'well-made play'.
- Companies included Jana Natya Manch (Janam): a Delhi-based company addressing workers' issues, questions of gender, democratic rights etc.; Kerala Sastra Sahitya Parishad (KSSP): mainly providing educational theatre and treating politically oriented issues in the southern state of Kerala. Many companies were allied to or inspired by the overarching Indian People's Theatre Association (IPTA).
- *Theatre of Roots*: single-authored plays drawing on traditional mythological material or indigenous performance forms to deal with contemporary issues of land-ownership, corruption, gender-relationships, inherited attitudes and behaviours.
- Dramatists include Girish Karnad, Habib Tanvir, Kavalam Panikkar, Chandrasekhar Kambar, Ratan Thiyam.
- *Social realism*: work centred on similar topics to those in the category above but articulated through contemporary characters and incident in a realistic format.
- Writers include Vijay Tendulkar, Mahasweta Devi, Satish Alekar, Mahesh Dattani.

A large proportion of these organisations, writers and directors originally had some association with IPTA and broadly left-oriented political positions; and the plays related to a wide spectrum of society from the rural poor and lower castes to the growing urban middle class, including issues of marginalisation and oppression by economic class, gender, conventional attitudes and separatist politics. Thus the formal and issue-related areas which Jana Sanskriti concerned itself with were similar to those found across the spectrum of post-Independence contemporary practice and debate found in *STQ* and in critical writing.

We'll see below that, even though Ganguly had had no formal the-atre training, both the focus of his work and the methodology which he began to develop could be seen to exhibit traces of many of these positions. In formal terms, all the three strands outlined above welded together Indian and non-Indian practice: 'agit-prop' messaging and political discussion, rural dance and music, 'western' realist conven-tions and so on. JS's work draws on local forms and global actor-training methodologies. Boal's 'gamesercises' model was itself a compilation and adaptation of many strands of existing practice, and in that sense lies within the trajectory of ('western') 19th- and 20th-century actor training (from Stanislavski via Copeau and Johnstone to Frantic Assem-bly) which both focuses increasingly upon bodily practice and aims to empower the actor as a creator. At the same time it's important to note that 'Jana Sanskriti ... went from activism to acting... from the beginning, theatre was a means for us to democratically intervene with people as activists' (Ganguly 2019: 371). It is the welding of acting and performance methodology with pragmatic political intent and intense engagement with spectator communities that characterises their par-ticular intervention into Indian theatre practice in the 20th and 21st centuries.

Seagull Theatre Quarterly (1996) has an account of a project with sex-workers in Kolkata on which JS collaborated, and reports on a subsequent performance-sharing and discussion which included women from their team and others from organisations elsewhere. The writers signal the personal and performative energy of the JS representatives: in discussion, '[w]hat impressed immediately was their confidence, their active participation, their questioning and verbal contribution' (Katyal 1996; 47); '[c]onsidering that they were participating in an event like this for the first time, they were invaluable contributors to the proceedings. They were sensitive, articulate and confident, they spoke from personal experience, they were living proof of the power of theatre activism' (53). And 'in performance one could see a lively sense of fun, humour, energy, an uninhibited enjoyment which the other troupes communicating social messages did not have' (48).

This suggests some distinctions from what is generally referred to as 'street theatre', which implies short message-oriented plays addressing economic and political issues, but with relatively limited dramaturgical sophistication. This is a charge not infrequently levelled at TO around the world, although neither in the global nor the Indian context is it by any means uniformly valid, and Boal is very clear that theatre demands the fullest spectrum of communicative channels and imaginative complexity. We will explore in more detail what steps JS have taken in performance and training to counteract this in following chapters. However, both in this respect and in the relationship to 'folk' performance, there are significant differences in JS's position. For one thing, Ganguly began by living, long term, in and with the communities from whom the first JS practitioners were drawn. Some of them were rural folk artists. So neither the political realities of life nor the accessibility and practicability of 'folk' forms was alien material or something that had to be acquired from elsewhere, as was sometimes the case with the relevance of workers' issues to middle-class intellectuals (Janam) or the 'retrieval' – or sometimes indeed 'reinvention' – of the 'traditional', as in the case of some of the proponents of Theatre of Roots or the earlier Madras (Chennai)-based founders of Bharatanatyam, India's best-known classical dance form. Issues and purposes, subject matter and artists, were already on site; and the latter emerged to join JS of their own volition because they found it useful as a channel through which to address their own concerns. As time went on and the processes they used developed, simple communication began to take on many further dimensions; but JS's work answered an immediately felt need and began to explore readily available means of articulating it.

SPECIFICS OF JANA SANSKRITI'S PERFORMANCE AESTHETIC

Jana Sanskriti combines the visual accessibility and intellectual interrogation of Boalian Image Theatre and Forum Theatre with leitmotifs and images drawn from Indian folk cultural forms, including well-known and resonant Baul songs and poems – and not infrequently, evocative poems about Bengal life by Rabindranath Tagore. This produces a theatre which resonates with the populations that make up their primary audience.

> The stories their plays tell across the rural landscape of Bengal are drawn from the lives of landless labourers, of wives in patriarchal homes and communities,

those marginalized from history, victims of *panchayat* corruption, party political violence, and victims of capitalist development.

(Mohan 2008: 5)

(More details will be given in Chapters Two and Three about the plays and the issues.)

The plays often use a repeated structural sequence of song and dance, narrative and plot, image and tableau, building up the tension in a scene to a striking frozen image, and releasing it in the dance or song which leads into the next movement. Jana Sanskriti groups also employ song as a starter, and many of them also use folk dance (e.g. the intricate, exciting and animated *kolattam* stick dance from Andhra Pradesh, sometimes referred by a local name as *kaathinaach*) to serve as an iconic 'warm-up' for performers and audiences alike. The structure of the play alternates exposition and encounter, frequently punctuated by various kinds of 'freeze' and leading to the open questions which are addressed to the audience, so '[t]he narrative structure ... is constantly broken during performance' (Iyengar 2001: 110), in a very 'Brechtian' invitation to interrogate the apparently 'given' narrative of social and political circumstances.

Ganguly had no contact with drama work before going to the villages, apart from seeing a few plays. As a child he had learned – and shown talent at – folk song and dance from various Indian states. In the villages he made contact with some folk artists, mainly from the Bengali forms called Jatra and Gajan; the villagers were largely familiar with stories and forms used in Jatra which they had seen regularly. Jatra, like other Indian 'folk' forms, uses elements from mythology but also relates them to contemporary settings; it includes distinctive music, song and quickfire, often rhymed, repartee; it is usually performed by artists who are paid per show.

Early on, Ganguly noticed that Indian folk performances have a number of ways of deconstructing the action. Heroes and gods are not necessarily shown as any more 'virtuous' than ordinary people: they can do stupid and venal things which produce catastrophic results. There is usually a 'clown' character and sometimes also a version of the Sanskrit *Sutradhara* ('the one who pulls the strings') – a kind of narrator-on-stage – both of whom have licence to satirise the powerful, elicit comment and involvement from the spectators, and speak in local dialects. We are already halfway to the Boalian 'Joker'; and Ganguly often says that if Brecht hadn't been born in Germany, he would have been Indian.

German playwright Bertolt Brecht (1898–1956) presented snapshots of contemporary social and political life before and during the Nazi period, often via parables or folk-tale format. He invited the audience to critique and analyse the action by repeatedly stopping, framing or interrogating it, using a narrator or commentator figure; a process which he called *Verfremdung*, or 'making strange'.

The essence of this making strange technique is embedded in Indian folk culture, as is the 'trickster'-like function of opening windows on different perceptions of 'reality'. So the incorporation of folk elements, particularly music, dance, masks and colourful costume, in addition to its ability to deliver different kinds of semiotic communication and connotation, consciously delivers the possibility of more complex, critical and egalitarian engagement.

For Ganguly, 'aesthetics' means how form influences the way you feel about and understand what you see. So it's a mode of relationship with the play and with yourself; the performance enables a recognition of the scope and acuity of intelligence in the spectators, which Party political cultural offerings, and sometimes conventional top-down theatre models, often failed to acknowledge. As we will see, this view also underpins many other dimensions of JS's work and characterises the whole nature of its practice.

In the journey towards evolving JS's distinctive style, several moments stand out. The recognition of folk theatre's potential is one; the next was an early performance of JS's second play, *Sarama* (1992), which presents successive incidents of violation and deprivation from a woman's life. Ganguly describes an encounter with women audience members after the show (Ganguly 2010: 16–19; 2009: 65–6) which crystallises the understanding that offering hopeful solutions is not enough: we can't do noble resistance to the boss's sexual demands, they said, because we have to feed our families. For those who know Boal's iconic stories, this insight recalls his 'Virgilio' moment (after a performance by Boal's troupe to peasant farmers advocating armed resistance to their oppressive landlords, Virgilio invited them to choose their weapons; Boal 1995: 2–3). As the women challenged the well-meaning optimism of the play's conclusion, Ganguly writes: 'I felt that the trees around me were moving, and the ground beneath my feet had suddenly begun to sway' (2010: 18). As a result, he rewrote the play and the new version asked the audience questions instead of proposing answers.

So this is about inhabiting the reality the audience lives, and ensuring that this audience is the source and substance of the dialogue about what to do about it. It's recognising that this form of theatre should be alert to the dangers of offering solutions rather than exploring predicaments. It's a learning moment about the relationship between play and audience, about the positionality of the participants, and about listening rather than prescribing. So it is right at the heart of Ganguly's key plank of practice, that what JS makes is Theatre *of* the Oppressed, not Theatre *for* the Oppressed.

These insights affect the way JS works with the key components of Forum, and will be returned to in Chapters Two and Four in terms of theory and practice. Essentially, they condition the way they:

- *deal with issues*: resist the temptation to 'fix it', avoid 'magic solutions', look to problematise and open up interrogation
- *view the 'Joker'*: as a 'referee' rather than a player, as a bridge between actors and potential spect-actors, as a stimulator and co-creator, not a director or author
- *construct their training*: find ways to pluralise perspectives, unpick 'backstories', physicalise the dialogic

Subsequently, Ganguly and other Jana Sanskriti members have been able to draw on such stories and access ways of materialising them precisely because they took note of this lesson and because their performance is combined with wide-ranging fieldwork. They operate constantly with an ear (and a couple of feet) to the ground. So this has manifested itself both in the structures of community involvement charted above, in their sensitivity to the dynamics of the situations people live in, and in the dramaturgy they employ.

ONGOING TRAJECTORIES

That work can be seen to have taken the company through three major parameters which have grown side by side: development of the methodology of training and community intervention; development of the core structures of the company; national and international interactions. All of them have grown in a more or less organic fashion, as each experiment and experience, which often included considerable problems, was part of a learning curve. So for instance the first encounters with TO practitioners began even before JS had become fully independent, but were a major factor in allowing the performers to become more confident, clear and coherent about their practice and its aims. Further, it began a process of international exchange which has gone on to incorporate a biannual festival, performances and workshops in many countries, productive relationships with scholars and researchers, students and practitioners from around the globe and across India, and a move into experimentation with new models of Forum and pre-scripted plays, some of them international 'classics' – all the while whilst sustaining and indeed expanding the activity outlined above across West Bengal and other Indian states.

I have already suggested that the first category can be understood as delivering a training both for actors and for spectators, who in the process become spect-actors and ultimately spect-activists. We will look in more depth at how some key exercises are used by Jana Sanskriti in Chapter Four, but an initial investigation is useful here. Because the issues JS plays deal with are rooted in the day-to-day experience of the people they work with, it is essential to find physical, rhythmic and direct ways of expressing situations. Often one of Boal's exercises (e.g. Colombian Hypnosis) is a good starting point, so that relationships between performers can be explored physically, and then interrogated for what they signal in terms of power dynamics. Jacques Lecoq, one of the best-known western theatre trainers of recent decades, emphasised that 'the body remembers'; and it can often articulate more succinctly and evocatively than words. Physical engagement gives the performers the chance to register what is happening to them in a situation, and to explore how they are affected emotionally and intellectually by it. JS's first actors – like many of the current teams, though now they include subsequent generations, some of whom are still students – mostly worked primarily with their bodies in daily life, as farmers, labourers, housewives; exercises and Image Theatre work came readily to them and could be readily understood by their audiences of peers. So pragmatically and dynamically, this was a productive way to go: the images and physicalised situations could be reflected on, explored, given voice or sometimes text, and developed into scenarios and scenes. In this process, the body becomes a source of signification, of expression and of provocation, in that it is part of a structure or a composite image which foregrounds and articulates a problematic situation or issue.

Different elements have gone into the mix at various times: coming across elements of Boal's training method and finding that it underpinned and gave a direction to what had already started to emerge; working with Jean-François Martel and the team from Paris who, somewhat bemusedly, followed Boal's request to land up on the outskirts of Kolkata and do some training workshops, introducing more Boal exercises which Ganguly studied carefully; working with other foreign practitioners including Boal's son Julian, and later with other practitioners from many countries who were fascinated by the work and offered input based on other approaches – improvisation, rhythm and sound, Rainbow of Desire. And all the time discussing the logics as well as the logistics, giving a shape to an emerging strategy in which the body becomes a more and more powerful creative site, encountering more and more strands of social and political complexity.

Chapters Three and Four will look at further dimensions of this. Boal's set of exercises and games were derived from many other existing models and adapted for purpose; many TO and Applied Theatre practitioners have similarly adapted them to their own circumstances and goals. Chapter Four will look at some of the specifics of how JS has developed their own versions whilst retaining the essential drive of Boal's vision. In terms of plays, Chapter Three, in addition to examining the form and content of typical JS plays which have been scripted through the lengthy co-creative activity of workshop (*Song of the Village*, *Where We Stand*, *Golden Girl* among them), will also interrogate why and how JS has in the past decade experimented with pre-existing scripted work from Africa and Europe, most recently Ibsen's *A Doll's House* in the context of attitudes to patriarchy in West Bengal. JS's practice is not static because neither its performers nor the contexts in which they work are static: in so far as the work is inextricably rooted in living circumstances it must also be alert to the necessity of adapting to that change.

In this way, JS has continually accommodated itself to different kinds of input and used them to extend and refine the ways it creates plays. Where and how these plays occur is also an important factor. Much of its work, as we have seen, is rooted in the villages of West Bengal, but even in doing it, JS often uses different kinds of activist engagement.

The parameters (and the numbers involved) of the events and processes organised by JS are wider than those of single performances.

RALLIES, MARCHES ETC.

These kinds of action, which occur as and when necessary, are ways of materialising solidarity, of reinforcing a sense of collective engagement, of making statements, of foregrounding key issues, of making people's active concern visible. Notable examples are i) two cycle rallies to Delhi (a distance of about 1500km) in support of a minimum contract for agricultural workers – 55 and 38 days, doing plays on the way (see Sima Ganguly in Da Costa 2010b: 40–1); ii) women marching to the police station to demand closure of illegal hooch operations, where activists also needed to counter a degree of police complicity (see Da Costa 2007: 300–2); similar large-scale representations targeting corruption by dealers in the ration-distribution scheme for those below the poverty line (BPL), or agitating for electricity connection to rural health centres.

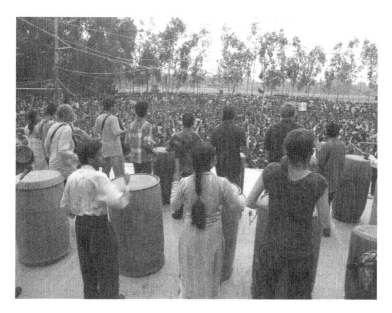

Figure 1.7 Audience at Muktadhara 4 event.

Photo: Jana Sanskriti

Other instances include thousands of people coming long distances with poor transport to Kolkata in 2006 to join with Augusto Boal to demand the right to culture for all; and festivals of JS work in the villages during the Muktadhara festivals (bi-annually from 2004), drawing crowds of between a few hundred and 10,000, many of whom are keenly aware of the Forum process and critically alert to all of its elements.

The range and remit of these events indicates that this is another dimension of doing theatre as politics: but always as more than spectacle. The numbers of attendees and the commitment they show is not in itself that unusual in the Indian context: there are areas in Delhi where people's demonstrations, marches and rallies take place regularly. But JS's events speak repeatedly and consistently to the same (if ever-expanding) constituency of supporters; and the events are only one part in a sequence of different kinds and levels of engagement. In none of these situations are the participants passive; far from it, many of them will walk long distances, take ferries or buses, help to construct, decorate or light the performance space, and then engage with the performance as spect-activists. 'Theatre is not enough' (Pramanik in Da Costa 2008: 1); because here theatre is the impetus to action of many kinds. The training or extended pedagogy builds towards and encompasses this spectrum of action.

MUKTADHARA FESTIVALS

Since 2004, JS has held biannual international festivals of TO. Muktadhara means 'many streams', implying the free flow of energy. Over the years, people from around 30 countries from across the globe have come to the festivals, which have in a number of ways also been factors in the material and intellectual extension of JS's own practice and its networking with practitioners across the globe. Not everyone who has come has been a TO activist; there have been many students, beginning to learn about this form of theatre and intrigued to take it further; there have been established practitioners from major TO groups – Formaat from Rotterdam in the Netherlands, TONYC from New York, Cardboard Citizens from London UK, CTO Rio from Brazil, CTO Maputo from Mozambique, Kaddu Yaraax from Senegal, TO Wien from Austria, TOP from Lille, France, groups from Bangladesh, Sri Lanka, Nepal, students and practitioners from Australia, Thailand, Iran, Iraq, Palestine, Germany, France; theatre teachers, scholars and researchers, practitioners who work in other but related modes. The festivals initially took place in Kolkata, which involved massive logistics to find lodging and arrange events. They have increasingly included phases located in the villages of the Ganges delta (the Sunderbans) where JS has established rural teams.

The pattern of events has shifted gradually over the years, but many of the central elements have remained. Although on one level such an event has always, given the nature of the participants, provided an important opportunity for people to meet, share ideas and forms of practice, and discuss principles and methodologies, JS has fundamentally conceived of it as a way of introducing its own model and method to the world.

The early Muktadharas 'allow Jana Sanskriti to experience itself as a collective of locally grounded struggles, sharing critiques and imagined strategies' (Da Costa 2007: 303). So they serve(d) as a moment of reflection of their own practice and process, whilst (increasingly) also opening out into an international dialogue about strategies and methodologies.

Thus in recent versions, at the core of the (two-week) event are firstly a practical induction to JS's way of working with sequences of exercises and developing scenarios, and secondly the opportunity to both practice and see the results of this in action and *in situ*, with a live audience. Initially this occurred in Curzon Park in central Kolkata, a well-known venue for political events and performance utilised among others by Badal Sircar, the most innovative in terms of location and format of Kolkata practitioners of the post-war decades. The JS central team, other Bengal teams and JS groups from elsewhere in India presented Forum plays which addressed major representative issues like the intercommunal violence in Gujarat in 2001 and the expropriation of land in Maharashtra, alongside pieces by the international participants. Impressive as this was, it became clear to the JS central team that this format was not fully getting inside JS's working practices. Seeing work from TO practitioners from a range of countries gave them the confidence to recognise the unique features of their own. Increasingly they became clear that it would be more useful to find ways of enabling international participants to experience as much of their methodology as possible. To present it as fully and clearly as possible, through practice and direct experience, would enable people to understand how and why it represented a particular mode of working with TO. This would still, of course, serve as a stimulus to comparative discussion and would, hopefully, cause foreign participants to interrogate their own practices in fruitful ways. But the focus of Muktadhara, especially in the years following Boal's death in 2009, has been on providing in-depth exposure to JS.

Two things in particular have occurred. First, the initial section of the festival has taken the form of a sequential workshop on 'Scripting the Play', delivered by Sanjoy Ganguly, which forms the basis of much of the material in Chapter 4. Other workshops by practitioners from a range of countries have often occurred alongside this, so the structure has both allowed people to experience how JS goes about the business of play construction and also to get some additional comparative input from leading practitioners: e.g. Till Baumann (Berlin), Peter Igelmund (Halle), Jean-François Martel (Lille), Luc Opdebeek (Formaat, Rotterdam), Birgit Fritz (TO Wien), Jale Karabekir (Istanbul), Tim Wheeler (Mind the Gap, Bradford), Julian Boal (CTO Paris, then Rio), Barbara Santos (CTO Rio, then Kuringa, Berlin), Ronald Matthijssen (Formaat, then TO Wien). The workshop culminates in the development of short Forum pieces in groups consisting of a mix of participants from different countries – i.e. the pieces are developed during the workshop and not pre-scripted or brought ready-made. It takes participants through the process of identifying issues, formulating a sequence of scenes representing one of them and leading to a problematic conclusion, and readying this proto-Forum play for performance.

A major development underpinning this section of the festival was where to site it. Kolkata, of course, offered a range of accommodation. So for the first three years, people were put up in a variety of hotels, discussion events were organised at various locations, and sometimes workshop activities could be provided. But the logistical demands for a very small company – administratively, three or four people at most in a single office with very basic equipment – were enormous: organising transport, lodging, events and, not least, looking after the health of participants in a very polluted city. It always risked being chaotic and incoherent – though it also managed to be exciting, stimulating and productive. So JS began to ask whether it would be possible to locate this first part in their home base of Badu. Workshops could take place in the centre (Girish Bhavan), which had been built in 1999, and in an adjacent mango orchard. So lodging was found in a variety of houses in the village of Badu nearby – which did however mean that for a few years there needed to be a reduction in the number of participants. Then, as a result of donations from local groups and international well-wishers, more work was done at Girish Bhavan. The initial single-storey building was extended to include simple but adequate accommodation, enough for about 30–40 people. Adding this to the village provision meant that the format could be cemented; and subsequently more funding allowed the construction of a third floor, to house the 'Augusto Boal auditorium', a small performance space with seating for about one hundred, inaugurated in 2015.

Here too then the process of development is not just about doing plays – it's about creating spaces in which that doing can occur, thinking about ways in which it can be extended, exploring how working methods can be effectively shared and paralleled in order to further discussion and exchange, about building quite materially – and much of it again with their own hands – and this work still goes on as JS reaches out to other organisations and institutions in the vicinity and beyond (the centre hosts events from local cultural and political groups, runs a restaurant service for the local college, and welcomes visitors of many kinds at regular intervals).

The second thing has to do with the location of the second part of the festival, the presentation and viewing of performances. Kolkata was accessible and working there was highly visible: good publicity

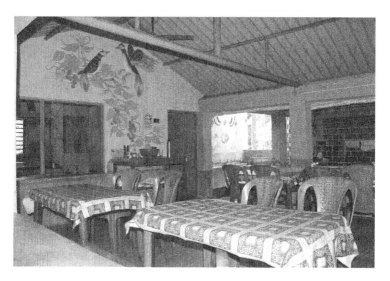

Figure 1.8 Dining area, Girish Bhavan.

Photo: Jana Sanskriti

for JS and TO – though the press tended to focus on the 'exotic' foreigners and ignore the remarkable fact that a largely non-funded group consisting mainly of workers in disadvantaged sectors had managed to acquire the international reputation which attracted those foreigners … But it's not where JS actually work. In some years, members of JS's regular audiences were – with considerable difficulty – brought to Kolkata. But this was not the same thing. People were not able to see the work in the field or get a sense of the conditions JS operated under. However, it seemed initially that it would be nearly impossible to provide lodging and food in the villages – which mostly lacked electricity and other basic services – for somewhere between 50 and 120 people. Gradually, a variety of creative solutions – always involving much hard work from many of JS's members in the field as well as the central team – enabled guests to stay in hotels and lodges and be bussed to events in villages. Visitors were entranced – sometimes in a rather naïve way, of course – with the simple life and the peace and beauty of the isolated locations; they were also able to see at first hand the ways in which spectators responded to Forum – not least because some of that theatre work was produced by the visitors themselves. To sit on a starlit night on plastic sheeting under an awning with over 2000 people focused intently on the illuminated stage specially constructed for the occasion, and to experience people from that audience getting up to intervene in the scenarios they were watching (most of which required translation between at least one and usually more languages, but which had all been developed through the preceding workshop so as to communicate clearly in a visual and rhythmic way) was a very powerful way to get access to how JS engages with the people who make it up.

Chapters Two and Three will explore further the ways in which some of these dimensions relate specifically to the construction and delivery of plays and to the activism which is initiated by them. What Muktadhara experiences like this have been able to do is to convey something of the network of relationships which constitutes JS to people from other continents and cultures. That raises all kinds of questions; it also speaks to JS's understanding that, for them, TO is more than an engagement with issues, more than a set of theatrical practices, more than a perspective on 'oppression'. It is all of these things. But it is also an attitude and a way of working which binds them together.

INTERNATIONAL CONTACTS AND RESEARCH

The relationships forged at Muktadharas have largely, though not exclusively, resulted in a growing body of researchers, scholars and practitioners who want to think critically and comparatively about JS's understandings and practices in relation to Applied Theatre, theatre and social change, TO and other related applications.

Students have done internships and written dissertations at BA, MA and PhD level; research projects in the last few years have been conducted by scholars from the Universities of Hyderabad and Leeds, and from the Institute of Social Science in Kolkata. Researchers from the USA, the UK, Austria and France have explored JS's work in books and articles, some of which are referenced in Chapter Two. All of this, plus the hundreds of Muktadhara participants over the years, many of them young TO practitioners or people who have been looking to apply theatre practice across a range of social and political contexts, has generated an atmosphere of continuous intellectual exploration and interaction. Since at the same time, members of core and satellite teams return frequently to the centre to rehearse, attend meetings, develop new projects and undergo further training in related (e.g. educational and medical) skills, as well as the intermittent presence of local artistic and political groups and networks, Girish Bhavan is nearly always very busy. Its activity encompasses a spectrum of practice, reflection, research and planning.

It was therefore a logical step to mark the vision and reach of this field by devising JSIRRI – the Jana Sanskriti International Resource and Research Institute – whose main purpose is to signal that JS and its various hubs of activity welcomes, and is open to collaborate with, projects and proposals of all kinds, both academic/theoretical and practical, relating to the use of theatre, performance and the arts in social, political and community contexts. JSIRRI's vision and mission statements declare that:

> JSIRRI's intention is to explore how Theatre of the Oppressed and related theatre and art forms can foster a culture of dialogue, strengthen participation and stimulate liberation by engaging with a wide range of disciplines and fields of work.

JSIRRI's open space extends an invitation to all those who want to propose projects, research into practice and/or offer resources in line with these goals, creating interdisciplinary dialogue and exchange to frame new challenges and nurture embodied and productive knowledge.

JSIRRI is not so much a physical entity as an invitation. It doesn't have funds or permanent staff – although members of the JS team collaborate on projects as appropriate, and it has to have minimal legal status under Indian law. It is able to publish books. In other respects it is largely invisible or informal, in that visits, projects, workshops etc. can be proposed by anyone at any time without needing 'official' sanctioning, providing that they are 'funding neutral' (i.e. cover any costs incurred by JS). It doesn't seek to promote a particular view of TO, though people who undertake projects will most probably be examining JS's methodology. It may or may not endure. But its existence is a useful way of circumscribing some of the dimensions of JS's international profile and its invitation to others to access its field of operations.

JS HQ is also frequently the site of extension activities which are more locally resourced but indicate another dimension of the attention JS pays to understanding the environment and issues it deals with: seminars with agricultural scientists, doctors, sociologists etc. in order to obtain expert input during the construction of plays, training with doctors for rural health workers, provision of space for an online network of West Bengal theatre practitioners. Outreach is also embedded into practice in these ways.

WHO?

JS is a team, a movement, a process, a model. It's everyone who contributes to this. However it is relevant to identify that it is the 'core team' which has been most concerned with directing the growth of this entity over the years. On one hand, because the organisation is its people. And on the other because to say a little more about them further highlights the way performance and practice operate in JS.

Sanjoy Ganguly dedicates his 2017 book to this core team. Their stories are sketched out by Dia Da Costa in *Scripting Power* (Da Costa 2010b: 10–19) and several of them (Sima Ganguly, Renuka Das, Pradeep Sardar, Pradeep Haldar, Pritilata Mondal, Kavita Bera, Chittaranjan Pramanik, Satyaranjan Pal) contribute essays to that book.

Here are some of the things they say about what brought them to JS, what spoke to them about its aims and methods and how they evaluate the results personally.

The first responses I report here are about independence of mind and self-worth and about a model of mutual respect. For Sima, it is the sense that culture and politics go inextricably together, the feeling that how JS do theatre offered a route to self-determination, the recognition that Jana Sanskriti '[doesn't] leave people to deal with the consequences of protesting', and the 'the sense of hierarchy is not … visible' (Da Costa 2010b: 40–4). Renuka puts it like this: 'Here, you can give some value, some importance to your own opinion. Here, you have space to work independently. No one is boss here. After coming here, I have seen a different world' (49). Pradeep Sardar finds that this kind of theatre 'addresses my mind's hunger' and is gratified by the recognition from spectators who were sceptical about the simple format that it did the same for them (76, 78).

Pritilal Mondal locates the link between methods and effects in terms of what might be called behavioural politics in the community: 'With the help of JS organizational strength and mobilization, the efforts of women in my village gathered much more strength. Theatre made us stronger' (83). This occurs in part because '[w]e're asking them to think about and debate questions that simply were not discussed in this way before' (84). Moreover, these debates refocus perspectives jn an important way: '[g]etting people things isn't the biggest thing in the world. This organization is thinking about their rights' (85).

Many of the core team articulate the need, as Priti does above, to offer alternative values to the advance of consumerism. So when Sima writes that as she grew as an actress, 'I learned to reflect' (39) and Renuka says 'I feel the change in my life. In my mind' (50), they echo the sense running through all these statements that their theatre activity is part of a nexus which extends them and the people they come into contact with both intellectually and politically. Chittaranjan and Satyaranjan highlight ethical and political insights which the work brought them. For Chitto, it is essential that words and actions should match (123): in contrast, in much party political activity he finds 'political terrorism' emanating from 'authoritarianism in the name of democracy' (125). Satya celebrates the fact that theatre has enabled discussion of questions and problems and meant that JS is taken seriously, demonstrating 'what Sanjoyda calls "theatricalisation of politics"'.

And within the organisation, though everyone has different skills and does different jobs, there is real equality rather than some kind of homogeneity (139).

Anjum Katyal, writing about Jana Sanskriti women performers/activists in *Seagull Theatre Quarterly*, has the following observations:

> There were no passive victims here, only fighters and survivors who had found a strength of their own—that message came through clearly. That this form of expression—theatre—gives them a powerful tool of communication and self-fulfilment was also very clear.
>
> (Katyal 1996: 48)

Most, indeed in some sense all, of JS's members have experienced some aspects of struggle (e.g. 'a Jana Sanskriti activist talked of how she had come out of a repressive family situation with an abusive father who had squandered everything on liquor; 45'). Although in many cases this was neither desired nor designed by them, what seems to unite them is the discovery that their communal practice provides a way of turning this into a positive drive, rather in the way that bringing an active awareness to bear upon problematic issues in a Forum session may lead to the possibility of new outcomes. And each of them has recognised fundamental aspects of the process which has run through the development of the company and its work.

This looks like one dimension in which Boal's desire to 'humanise humanity' is working. We will also pick this up further in Chapter Two with reference to a reflection on what 'self' might mean in this kind of context and some of the ways in which Ganguly understands the process of interactive relationship which JS supports.

Although there are plenty of actors and other kinds of performers who have long careers, and many people who have worked in TO or other kinds of activist theatre over decades – many running companies or organisations – it is pretty rare for a performance company of any kind to retain a substantial group of members for this long (other examples might be Eugenio Barba's Odin Teatret, The Wooster Group, or Forced Entertainment). So the JS 'core team' is an unusual example. Around a dozen of them have been with JS for well over two decades, and have taken on increasing levels of responsibility, including creating, training and running their own teams, which in some cases include children of the first group. Over the years they have expressed doubts and disagreements, worried about the future of JS, and yet remained a part of its 'family', which is a term both they and Ganguly often use. This model might not be reproducible elsewhere, but it is worth reflecting on its key components. Many of them have been outlined in the preceding section and some ramifications of these will be explored in the next one. Perhaps the most important is the suggestion that 'relationship' – however you might want to define that notion – is a key factor to everything they do.

It's also important to say a little more about Sanjoy Ganguly.

This series has to date dealt with individual directors, play-makers and actor-trainers. Some of them (Barba, Jacques Copeau, Jerzy Grotowski, Tadeusz Kantor, Joan Littlewood, Ariane Mnouchkine) have worked extensively with a particular group or groups of actors; others (Pina Bausch, Konstantin Stanislavsky, Jacques Lecoq, Vsevolod Meyerhold, Augusto Boal, Peter Brook, Michael Chekhov, Rudolf Laban, Barba again) have put their mark on a particular training process or performance methodology. Ganguly is an ensemble leader, an actor-trainer, a director, a playwright and an activist. In many of these dimensions his work reaches out to an extent comparable with or greater than that of these figures. Like many of them he is also a seminal thinker who refashions understandings of his field and translates them into repeatable action. He has an international reputation across the globe both within TO, as one of the major points of reference of practice and of the extension of Boal's legacy, and as a teacher and workshop leader who has regularly contributed to work at many institutions. In the Indian context he receives much less public recognition; but he has produced a quantity and quality of work which is comparable to other leading directors and writers, and has additionally written clearly and comprehensively about his work in a variety of publications.

Chapter Two will examine further and elucidate some of the key ideas which he articulates in his writing. Chapter Three looks at some of his plays and directing methodology. Chapter Four will work with aspects of his training trajectory.

There are many reasons to suggest that the name Sanjoy Ganguly should figure in the title of this book alongside that of Jana Sanskriti, the company and activist movement which he has envisioned, shaped, nurtured and sustained. If it does not, it is because, in spite of the significance of all the things mentioned above, what he has constructed is above all a densely interwoven and fiercely collectivist set of relationships in which theatre process becomes the weft of artistic, social, political and ethical practice. Even so, it's important to underline that Jana Sanskriti is in many ways indistinguishable from Sanjoy Ganguly.

WRITING ABOUT JANA SANSKRITI

OVERVIEW

This chapter aims to refocus the 'who/where/what/why' of Chapter One by looking at how Sanjoy Ganguly and other writers have positioned and evaluated Jana Sanskriti's practice. To set that up, the chapter starts with a condensed summary of the main tactics, attitudes and principles which characterise JS's practice. It then goes on to examine in some detail the central features of Ganguly's thinking about the work, mainly derived from his 2010 book *Jana Sanskriti, Forum Theatre and Democracy in India,* and concludes by presenting some ways in which both Ganguly and other writers have evaluated the outcomes of that work. As Chapter One has shown, JS works in specific geographical, social and political contexts. In so doing, it uses some elements common to other similar practice, but works with them in particular ways.

KEY PARAMETERS OF JANA SANSKRITI'S PRACTICE

Forum events, workshops, exercises and training, as JS deliver them, are about bringing together people and practice. The what is also a how. It is what you work with and how you work. JS use components of much socially engaged theatre practice: people, plays, exercises,

DOI: 10.4324/9780429288753-2

principles of working in groups, strategies to develop collective creativity. But during the course of working over the years, those components began to shape a particular mode of operation. The methods and principles derived from them emerged during the course of JS's engagement with the people who make up their audiences and activists. One vital element is their growing understanding that, in addition to its specific rooting in daily social realities and its impact on the political circumstances which frame them, the work they are engaged in can also be seen as a *practice of relationship*. This insight illuminates the threads which run through all dimensions of their activity: making plays, developing a movement, activating people, taking care of the spectrum of needs and responsibilities which this entails. It is in this sense, as well as in the performances they create and the effects they produce, that they represent a major example of contemporary performance practice and a distinct and perhaps radically significant way of doing politics. Some of the main planks of their endeavour which have been identified or suggested in the previous chapter are:

'process not entity':

- working as a collective
- establishing a methodology of exchange
- developing responsive nodes of activism
- listening and responding to local needs
- scripting and rescripting stories
- training activists and service providers
- shifting habits and customs
- recalibrating committee processes

'thinking with the heart':

- recognising, valuing and nurturing individual and shared capacities
- engaging multiple knowledges
- inhabiting complex personal and interpersonal sociopolitical structures
- providing opportunities to play, create and reflect
- acknowledging and working with difficulties; valuing what goes wrong
- stirring up gendered assumptions; challenging internalised mindsets
- relocating the shared community; resisting class and caste division

'theatreing politics':

- animating and problematising issues; embodying and dynamising analysis and action
- exposing corruption, duplicity, manipulation
- staging resistance to monologue and indoctrination; ironising and deconstructing hierarchies
- energising local cultural resources
- reforming local democratic structures
- transforming public space

As JS has grown into this work and discovered its methodology in and through it, it has had to face challenges. Some of the forms they take are:

dramaturgical: finding an appropriate model for the task, the personnel, the cultural and historical/political moment; avoiding reductionism and agit-prop

methodological: discovering how to work with the target communities; adapting Boal to local conditions; overcoming logistical difficulties (funding, travel, communication etc.); finding a way to make 'poor theatre' both dialogically effective and aesthetically stimulating

ethical and political: negotiating dangers of instrumentalism; overcoming internal and external alienation; establishing practices of democratic participation within the organisation at all levels; negotiating complex political contexts; countering ingrained prejudices and antagonisms; finding channels, both within and outside existing political structures, to engage with local issues and needs.

For JS the practice of performance is:

- a political psychophysiology of theatre
- a conscious act of resistance to fundamental neoliberal and doctrinaire assumptions
- a reconfiguring and recombining of the aesthetic, the material, the political, the ethical and the spiritual
- an ecology, which realigns the relationship of people, spaces, and modes of being and doing, within a specific geographical and social context

Within and beyond TIE/DIE (Theatre/Drama in Education) drama and theatre is recognised as delivering skills and nurturing values which are relevant beyond the stage or circumscribed event. There is also a long history of plays and practice which address social and political contexts and issues. Much recent scripted theatre in India and across the world does this excitingly, inventively and intelligently, although its effects are relatively difficult to quantify.

Jana Sanskriti's practice, strongly allied to much of this spectrum, is a distinctive form in its own right. It is certainly far more than 'street theatre'; it is also not just 'political theatre', but rather a politics of theatre and a challenge to the mutual definition of both. JS's work relates directly to everyday political realities, to social interactions, to communication and pedagogy, to a practice of aesthetics in a wide sense, to behavioural change and impacts in community structures. It also offers a significant contribution to the understanding of how and why theatre *works*, and how and why theatre *matters*.

This book is about 'practice' and 'performance'; and the first chapter has demonstrated that JS's work has fundamentally to be seen in these terms, as something that takes place in and through bodies, through all the ways in which they access, process and perform experience and response, as a spectrum of material encounters with places, people and the tactile conditions in which they live and work. It is also how bodies are changed by that process, and how they accommodate and use those changes in their relationships to these conditions. However, one of the essential components of the practice that JS delivers, both in Forum events themselves and in their repetition and follow-up, is the alternation of action and reflection; they interact and propel each other forward, as Ganguly continually emphasises. One is of little value without the other. So this chapter aims to point to some of the ways in which that reflection has materialised, both in Ganguly's positioning of the work and in other responses to it; and to continue some of the explorations that it sets in motion.

TOWARDS CONSCIOUSNESS WHICH DESIRES CHANGE: SANJOY GANGULY'S *JANA SANSKRITI, FORUM THEATRE AND DEMOCRACY IN INDIA* (2010)

Ganguly's two books (the one identified above, plus the 2017 *From Boal to Jana Sanskriti: Practice and Principles*) are the chief source for much of the material about JS's history, development, principles and practice. All other writing about JS – with the exception of one book, referenced in the last part of this chapter – appears in chapters, articles, dissertations and theses, and is cited either in this chapter or the previous one, in relation to the specific areas it focuses on. Apart from the short chapters in Dia Da Costa's *Scripting Power*, translated by her from Bengali and referred to in Chapter One, there is no published writing by other members of JS.

Jana Sanskriti, Forum Theatre and Democracy in India (Ganguly 2010), is a mixture of anecdote and reflection which describes key moments from JS's work and from workshops he conducted in India and abroad; the book uses them to think about the ethics and strategies of JS's practice by comparing it with that of Boal and others. Ganguly is not concerned with charting a clear historical sequence, but with showing *what* he and JS do and explaining *why* they do it like that. He is also perhaps more interested in giving a feel for the work than in pursuing a through-line of argument, since what is paramount for him is the *attitude* which you bring to it; that attitude is underpinned by personal and political convictions which are frequently explicit in his writing. The book addresses key themes and issues of JS's work, though Ganguly's writing, like his teaching, does not always follow a strictly sequential course. Instead, it tends to move in circles or spirals, using incidents and stories to illustrate important aspects, beginning to reflect on them and then returning in a later section or chapter to approach the same issue from a different perspective. The method is like JS's ongoing pedagogical process across repeated Forum events, meetings, and the passage of time: opening space for assimilation and reflection, allowing thought to move to new levels and leaving time for insights to dawn. For that reason it is useful to pick out key markers of this trajectory, because it parallels the development of JS's practice and shows how it relates to the categories outlined above. (Much of what appears in his second book, *From Boal to Jana Sanskriti*, is dealt with in Chapter Four, since it relates to exercises which JS use.)

Some of the main junctions of Ganguly's discussion are:

- recognition of new circumstances (physical and social)
- awareness of the potential of the aesthetic to impel 'new thinking'
- analysis of how that thinking can be understood and developed in the exchange and interaction of Forum, in the context of confronting real social and community challenges
- consideration of how the understanding of 'self' is consequently refocused, and why that is significant in the context of the work that JS do

The next sections will outline these and then ask how they relate to the kind of theatre practice JS delivers, mainly by looking at examples of how it has worked in specific situations.

***

Ganguly starts the story of JS with his personal journey as a young Party worker committed to finding out the reality of the conditions most of the people he aimed to help had come from. You could say that this represents an exploration of how to 'perform' politics, by first discovering directly how it was operating *in situ*. So he sets the scene of the physical experience of the early days, first in Midnapore block on the west bank of the Hooghly/Ganges river. The village is a 90-minute walk from the station; in the rainy season it takes twice as long, as 'the rains ... make the clayey soil dangerously slippery'; worse, near the villages the mud is mixed with excrement as there are no toilets and it is dangerous to go too far into the fields (Ganguly 2010: 8). There are no doctors, no electricity; three of the seven people who had come from the city returned there after a while. The physical specificity of the situation is not only descriptive: it is a means for Ganguly to identify how he engaged with a new kind of reality. Writing about 'the people' with whom he went to work in the villages, Ganguly says: '[t]he politics taught by the Party highlighted their economic condition, but neglected [their] human qualities. I had a vague idea about empowerment earlier. I am beginning to think differently now' (Ganguly 2010: 16).

What triggered this awareness was firstly, *living* in the environment with them (experiencing a condition which is both physical and material, and also much more than that); and secondly discovering unexpected resources which they used to deal with it. Music, he writes, 'wafted in the air'; folk forms brought him into contact with young performers, and '[g]radually I found myself being attracted by the entire concept of performance and its rich possibilities' (12). 'Performance' thus comes to signify a spectrum of modes of understanding and acting which are based in openness, fluidity and the potential of change. Ganguly recalls that his father opened some of this combination of art, politics and human relationship to him; but being embedded in new locations and having to face new challenges in daily life cements and expands that vision for him. Aesthetics isn't a philosophical concept; it's a mode of living in the world and responding to what it presents.

Ganguly characterises the recollection of this period as 'going back to the source'. That source is embodied experience, and by writing about it in this way, he is trying to locate a new way of being which underlies the rest of the journey and emerges as a new kind of thinking. In other words, rediscovering the source means getting in touch with the condition in which thinking can change. Ganguly says that 'to lose touch with the source is to me a kind of death' (ibid: 8), because it means losing that capacity to change. His metaphor is not a mere poetic flourish; it is part of what I have called 'thinking with the heart' in the opening section, which feeds into 'providing opportunities to play, create and reflect'.

So he begins to work with young people, some of them folk performers, and create scenes of village life which eventually coalesce into JS's first play, *Gayer Panchali* (*Song of the Village*). As he does so, another series of insights emerges.

In 1985, before he had come across Boal's work at all, JS composed a manifesto which said: 'We will not perform on the stage, because that creates inequality' (Ganguly 2010: 23), and points out that usually in indigenous Indian forms 'the performers and the spectators sit at the same level'. When, 'around 1990–91', Ganguly first encountered Boal's work – he read part of *Theatre of the Oppressed* – it helped JS to identify that, although the rural oppressed they were addressing were participating in the work in several ways, they didn't have equal status. Thus for Ganguly, Boal's writing 'opened up a new horizon' (ibid: 22), and 'coming into contact with Augusto Boal's thinking was certainly a moment of rebirth for Jana Sanskriti' (23). (Boal sent Ganguly a copy of *Games for Actors and Non-Actors* in 1992.) In this context, as Ganguly recounts, JS developed greater collectivity of input, began to create the network of committees and local organisation, fostered discussion amongst both men and women and moved towards the iconic play *Shonar Meye* (*Golden Girl*), which presents stages from a woman's life arising from a hundred images created by village women in workshops (25).

Ganguly records that during this period, the JS performers began to develop a sense of their own status, to feel that they had 'a new identity' and were able to 'disturb those in power' (14); he recognises the strength, resilience, 'generosity and energy' of the people they were working with (15); and writes about the 'lightbulb moment' of the challenge by women spectators after a performance of *Sarama* in Bir-bhum district, which triggered a major rethink and shifted their work from theatre *for* the oppressed towards theatre *of* the oppressed (see Chapter Three for a fuller description of this and the play).

Alongside this comes the recognition that the practice of Forum is the site of an encounter for both actors and spectators, moving them to identify and critique the roles they play on and offstage. It offers spect-actor and actor the chance to 'be touched for a moment by a different kind of consciousness' (32–3). Spectators are challenged to perceive their own behaviour in the scenarios they are watching; actors may realise that they do not always escape the traps they portray on stage.

Thus Ganguly uses the opening chapter of his book to pick out fundamental ingredients of what will become the JS methodology, which coalesce into an underlying dynamic principle which informs all aspects of the work. He calls this 'a consciousness which desires change, which is an expression of empowerment' (35). This new kind of consciousness, which is essential for real political change, is disclosed in Ganguly himself and in those with whom he works by the operation of 'theatre':

> Theatre is not just a performing art. It is much more. Theatre hides within itself answers to questions such as who am I, what is my strength etc. Theatre is something with the help of which a new revelation takes place every day, every minute. Boal says theatre is a discovery, from which we learn about ourselves.
>
> (Ganguly 2010: 39)

That is to say, the awareness and agency which are stimulated are both aesthetic and critical, both empowering and challenging, and what they set in motion is action.

MOVING TOWARDS A NEW POLITICS

Theatre, then, is a way to do politics which takes into account different dimensions of the human – and may thus impel a new kind or concept of 'politics'. The situation in which JS works is in many ways an extreme case of 'democratic deficit', in which, even if they live in a so-called democracy, people feel that they have little power over the actions of leaders; and this is likely to be increasingly the case towards the bottom end of the economic or social spectrum, disallowing the possibility of critique, intervention, the framing of alternative scenarios, transition or transformation. Extreme also because in West Bengal, structures of governance down to village level are dominated by political parties, and because at the same time the overarching framework of procedure, in spite of 30 years of avowedly left-wing (CPM/LFG) rule, has come to reflect capitalist 'definitions of value ... which encourage the formation of certain types of relations among people, nature and things' (Da Costa 2010b: 618). Class (and to some degree caste) has compounded the situation: 'In a class-divided society information is capitalised within a class. Some people have more information, more knowledge, some people have little' (Ganguly, unpublished draft for speech, 2016).

As we've seen in Chapter One, the CPM's use of culture tended to reinforce this situation. It is one in which some people get to speak *for* others and define the terms in which the speaking occurs and the values which govern daily life are set; whilst others are regarded as digits in the 'vote-bank' accounts of political parties, to be persuaded or corralled into ticking the right boxes at election times. Since the CPM's loss of power, the situation has if anything become more convoluted, although many areas with strong JS presence are typified by both cultural and political co-operation across the divides and the Digambapur region has won an award as the best-run *panchayat* in India.

So where does that co-operation start? To overcome the 'politics of divide and rule' and '[i]n order to establish equality, first recognise the intellectual ability of the people. If there is an intellectual equality, then true equality is just a matter of time' (Ganguly 2010: 121). As a consequence of this recognition, 'JS refuses the assumption that the middle-class and the poor have no choice but to accept the status quo' (Da Costa 2010b: 625). Theatre thus becomes the space and the form of a push back, and its operations signal that 'struggles to access and control the means of representation are a battle for citizenship' (Da Costa 2007: 316). It enables people to construct their own agendas; they 'are no longer just implementing agencies of the policies created by the system' (Ganguly 2017: 86). More specifically, says Ganguly:

> Theatre of the Oppressed provides a means of addressing this deficit and delivering Marx's original intentions, which include the development of holistic human capacities (thought + feeling + action) and the critical evaluation of the structural and historical factors of people's economic and social conditions.
>
> (Ganguly 2010: 138)

According to Sameera Iyengar, JS's political goal lies in 'bringing out the capacity for responsible thought and action, for agency, which is latent in every human being' (Iyengar 2001). Both in their group process and in performance, they seek to create such a 'political space': but the feeling for that space has first to be located within the physical, emotional and cognitive functioning of individual people, bearing in mind also that 'the individual is not isolated from the society' (Ganguly 2010: 125).

Ganguly's shift in thinking arises from immersive experience and informs a practice of relating to and working with others. It is a kind of affective and relational cognition, which perceives the network of connection between thought, feeling and action, and between cultural and material context and interpersonal behaviour. This is how Ganguly begins to see the power of theatre. Its aesthetic qualities, as Boal recognised, are what enables it to engage wider dimensions of knowledge and expressivity, to give credence to a more extended understanding of human capacity: in this sense, aesthetics is also a politics. This is particularly relevant in strata of society, like those JS works in, which have rarely been credited with these attributes.

Theatre is also fundamentally interaction. Between feeling, understanding and expressing; between creators of different kinds; between actors; between performers, performance and audience. The well-known trajectory from Brecht to Boal attempts to stimulate this process further in both actors and spectators; firstly by inviting critical reflection, and secondly by encouraging physical and vocal intervention in the performance as a 'rehearsal for revolution'.

As Chapter One has outlined, recognising that everyone has the capacities to do this, and offering the space to do it, are at the basis of JS's work. As everything is set in motion, acting and action become a form of deploying agency – the agency first of recognising feelings and intentions, then of expressing, working together, understanding, negotiating and transmitting. It's not just that in performing, people move, speak, sing, get up, open themselves and their faces to an audience; though it is all that. It's also that they thereby attain a different status, a way of being, a sense of self: within themselves *and* in relationship with others.

So a shift in thinking leads to a way of performing self and relationship as a conscious personal and collective response to the closing down of spaces for democracy and agency. It helps to identify that JS perceive theatre as a way of learning together how to do this. This mode of operation is already opening up space, as it were, both within and beyond the usual understanding of 'self'. In the process, 'non-actors' become actors, of various kinds and potentialities; and actors become more alert, inventive and extensive in their acting and their action.

FROM SELF-DISCOVERY TO COLLECTIVE AGENCY THROUGH THEATRE

In Chapter Two of his book (pp. 41–54), entitled 'Boal's theatre: The recognition of resource', Ganguly uses a couple of stories told by Boal and a lengthy account of working with some of his exercises to explore how people can begin to see themselves differently; Chapter Three, 'Boal's poetics as politics', engages with fundamental attitudes towards self and others by paralleling Boal's thought with that of Indian and western thinkers, and beginning to chart a vision of politics which goes beyond the situation Ganguly encountered in his early involvement with the CPM. The time he is writing about here is roughly the 1990s, when JS had taken on board the principles of TO and was experimenting with many of Boal's exercises in training, as well as using Forum in performance.

Ganguly quotes the Bengali sage Sri Ramakrishna's gloss on a story from the *Puranas*, about a tiger which didn't know what it was until shown its reflection in a pond: 'a teacher is a facilitator who helps you to understand yourself' (2010: 41). He then retells Boal's version of a Chinese folk-tale, in which Xua Xua starts to question the nature of identity, and points out that for Boal, the beginning of introspection is the genesis of theatre: 'she becomes her own spectator, watching the different thoughts and actions that she herself is carrying out' (43). Subsequently, he refers to another story from Boal, about a domestic worker called Mary, who gets to act in a play. In the mirror in the green room, she sees herself 'for the first time as a woman'. Ganguly comments: '[h]ere we witness the identity of the girl transforming in her own consciousness, from a housemaid to that of a woman, a human being' (54). So in all of these parables, as Ganguly interprets them, we are in the presence of a new way of seeing yourself and a recognition of innate capacity, which he identifies as fundamental components of the process of theatre.

In between these stories is an account of working through an exercise – derived from *The Rainbow of Desire* and *Games for Actors and Non-Actors* – with a boy whom Ganguly names Bakam (43–53). We'll look at this again in the context of Rainbow work in Chapter Four, but the essential point here is that the exercise is a step on the way for Bakam to experience, and perhaps resolve, 'the contradictions of will and desire within himself' (52). In presenting and vocalising images of Bakam's desire to negotiate his oppressive situation and the forces ('cops in the head') which constrain him, the other participants provide support and are able to reflect back to him the different impulses he experiences.

Having thus identified the ability to interrogate the self and to begin to reshape it as basic to theatre practice, in the next chapter Ganguly extends the implications of this as a pedagogy, as a method of political and philosophical enquiry, and as the groundwork for 'human sympathy'.

At the centre of the argument are two key observations from Boal. The first is his reflection on the Virgilio incident referred to earlier (p. 35). Recognising the shortcomings of his troupe's stance (singing 'let us spill our blood' but immediately clarifying that their weapons were not real and they could not actually join the peasants' revolt), Boal recalls the celebrated revolutionary Che Guevara's dictum: *solidarity means running the same risk* (cit. Ganguly 2010: 59, italics in original). Thus, Ganguly emphasises, for Boal, 'becoming a true artist' requires 'the integration of thought, words and action' (59). A couple of pages later, Ganguly highlights the fact that the human being 'is at the centre' of Boal's theatre, and possesses 'the three basic qualities of being sympathetic, passionate and rational' (2010: 61) That, he suggests, is in large measure why Boal's vision of 'humanising humanity' is undertaken through theatre.

These then are the expansive and relational criteria for the extension of human being around which the chapter circles. That is also why its main thrust is the need to expand the understanding of politics to include a 'poetics', which might be glossed as an emotionally intelligent and generous practice of making sense of one's world. Ganguly underscores his argument by linking Socrates' dialectical method and Paulo Freire's pedagogy of exchange between teacher and learner (ibid: 62–3); both recognise innate capacities for rational debate and sympathetic understanding as integral to all humans. Plato has Socrates promote 'the culture of asking questions' (63); Freire underlines 'the natural talents' in humanity (62).

The chapter opens with a story – perhaps apocryphal, but personalised by Ganguly – about a doctor who was prepared to listen to a suicidal patient on the phone in the middle of the night. The next day she tells him that what stopped her committing the act was not his knowledge, but his *attitude*, which, says Ganguly, showed not only 'a genuine desire to save life', but, crucially, 'a relationship of mutual respect and heart-felt warmth … really listening to each other' (57).

These are qualities which Ganguly looks for in his own practice of making theatre with communities, and in the fundamentals of Boal's work. In Boal and Freire, he sees 'a theory and practice of education which respects the knowledge of the common masses and the dignity of the oppressed' (62), and which is also profoundly Marxist without being doctrinaire (because empathetic engagement, questioning, debate and reciprocity are at its core). Seeing yourself, recognising similarities and distinctions with others, being open to engagement and dialogue are key components of the kind of theatre he wants to make.

Paulo Freire expresses the need for education to be based in dialogue and exchange, and suggests that by 'increas[ing] their capacity to enter into dialogue not only with [others] but with their world, [people] become "transitive"'. He goes on to claim that 'transitivity of consciousness' makes people 'permeable' (Freire 1976b: 17).

We could say that Ganguly himself first experiences this transitivity in his own encounter with life in the rural villages, as described above; he further emphasises in this chapter that '[i]t is through establishing personal relationships and bringing people face to face with themselves that human development can happen' (63). The process of dialogic exchange is embedded into Forum and extended into the long-term pedagogy of exchange which JS operate in its work with communities, in which the practice of doing and thinking alternate over a long period of time to produce ongoing and continuous change. Hence it is the result of both body-centred theatre work and intellectual exercise, both of which are a kind of dialogue. Changing the *way* we think is not a dilettante form of introspection. It is a political necessity which requires practice.

Empowering the 'self' to participate in that critique, as Ganguly presents it here, is facilitated by Boal's dramaturgy, which involves 'the interaction of the senses', and 'minutely reflecting on an experience from as many perspectives as possible' (69–70). This activation of body and intellect in alternation is reflected in JS's training and practice. Knowledge is created and transformed through the interplay of experience and analysis (or, we could say, action and reflection), as Ganguly signals (68); Boal, says Ganguly, 'elevated the art of knowledge by making it a public and collective process of exchange and debate through the medium of theatre' (72).

To that should be added Ganguly's essentially Boalian understanding of aesthetics:

> Aesthetics is a dialectical process of knowing – it is experience + new data > synthesis, i.e. it is organic (structural) and it produces a feeling of increased oneness and coherence. Thus subsequently this feeling drives the desire (will) to make relationships between things, people and situations ... The aesthetic as a mode of knowing is thus both sensitive and volitional. We experience, we recognise, we desire, we act, we create and we cohere.
>
> (Ganguly 2017: 141–2)

This chapter thus identifies the essential components of both 'human sympathy' and the 'open mind', and explores how in Boal's vision of theatre and JS's practice, they can lead to critical competency and collective action.

COLLECTIVE THINKING: MODES AND CONTEXTS

So building on the extension of the understanding of 'self', and on the ways it interacts with others in constructing and delivering the process of Forum, leads to a 'politics of collective thinking' (2010: 119–26), which is developed in the course of addressing real-life situations.

Forum is a mechanism by which collective thinking is practised and strategised. Ganguly says that JS's practice 'establish[es] an equilibrium between the actors and spectators ... [who] watch ... analyse, comment ... and discuss solutions they can implement' (2010: 66–7). And the purpose of Forum, in Ganguly's view, is not just to drive straight towards solutions, but rather – in the work of both the Joker and the actors – 'to create confusion, contradictions, and some convictions' (Ganguly 2017: 94). Boal himself described this as manifesting 'conflict, contradiction [and] confrontation' (Boal & Soeiro in Howe et al. 2019: 67). The perspectives and positions of protagonist, antagonist and other actors in the scenario are interrogated as fully as possible: '[d]ifferent theses may arise', but '[t]he most important thing is that we are all in transition, we are ready to be changed following a positive conflict of thought' (Ganguly 2010: 120). Theatre becomes a space for critical thought; Forum is 'a method and concept for politics', in which actors and spectators together 'undergo an intellectual exercise that empowers them for future action' (ibid).

For Ganguly, being a performer (actor or spect-actor) in Forum is also a way to become 'the spectator of your own action' (Ganguly 2010: 27, 32, 35). The term spectator here implies the quality of criticism, and also applies to the audience in general, since they are engaged in observing, identifying and interrogating situations, actions and outcomes which they recognise as pertaining to their own reality. Da Costa suggests that in viewing and participating in JS's practice of Forum, it is possible to become a 'spect-actor of history' – in other words to frame oneself within a social, historical and political moment and begin to reflect upon its constituents. Such a spect-actor is '[o]ne who engages in constant critical play on and offstage by upsetting the assumed boundaries between fiction and reality in order to construct social change' (Da Costa 2010b: 16). The 'safe space' of 'fiction' is thus seen as generating the play of critical thought, which arises in the exchange between people, perspectives and power dynamics. Ganguly makes it clear that this interplay is essential: '[i]nternal revolution does not take place ... in isolation ... [i]t requires a collective force ... self-introspection is the reflection of thinking from collective perspectives' (2010: 127).

Critical thinking and Forum methodology: the journey to collective action

- Critical thought identified: Forum emerges from and challenges Plato and Brecht on theatre as dialogue; it overtly positions critical thought as a political act: interrogating the 'given', recognising alternative perspectives, negotiating social and interpersonal space
- Critical thought set in motion: Forum stimulates critical analysis of the structural causes of specific issues; it seeks to extend the vision from the particular to the general
- Critical thought embodied: spect-actor interventions activate the performance space for actors, spect-actors, Joker and audience (the performance event becomes a critical space)

- Critical thought dynamised, transported and negotiated: the performance as gift gives rise to reciprocity from the community; then to ongoing analysis and action/reflection in committees and beyond (the event extended as durational practice)
- Critical thought realised: as collective rational action; onstage action translated into activism beyond the stage: the community or society becomes theatre in action

This trajectory can also be understood as the enhancement of different levels of 'deliberative' action, in the sense of developing the confidence and capacity to embrace 'the decision that life can have room for decisions' (Julian Boal in Da Costa 2010b: 118) and then taking this forward into forms of collective decision-making and action. The enhancement of thinking and feeling which emerges from participation in JS's processes can also help to address 'undercover' forms of structural oppression (instances of invisible power and communal/'traditional' beliefs that are largely unconscious and internalised by social norms, rather than explicitly intentional); and to pursue strategies that enable people to better recognise and challenge these boundaries. The whole process is a way of learning how to 'strategize collectively' (Lynne 2014: 7). As JS's practice bears out, this sometimes involves changing quite radically the interim decisions taken after a Forum and the actions which result from them; it is an ongoing critiquing process.

That's why the Joker's job in a Forum session is to help the spectators and spect-actors to recognise and negotiate 'difficult' moments, as well as doing it him/herself. It's another step in the ongoing pedagogy and it is also a sign of the way things are working in the session. In addition to difficultating, Ganguly emphasises that the Joker needs to understand the importance of the collective. This means recognising the wisdom of the assembled company and the potential which resides in the plurality of its contributions – even, or particularly, when they don't immediately seem to 'fit' with what the Joker might think is useful; it marks an openness which frees up the ability to learn – echoing the way Freire conceived of the mutual exchange between teacher and learner. As we will see in Chapter Four, this is also a vital element of workshop practice for JS. Ganguly is adamant that the Joker's main function is to assist the 'game' to go on by facilitating the interaction between all participants. It's 'like refereeing in football', in which the players, not the referee, 'score the goals' (Ganguly 2017: 103–4).

For Clément Poutot, TO renders public space 'civic, propositional, [and/or] oppositional', through plays which can be defined as 'offensive, defensive [and/or] reflexive' (Poutot 2015: 368). What happens in public space usually tends to follow rules of procedure and hierarchy, but Forum explicitly reshapes these. In other words, the dramaturgy is the medium and the message, as it is a set of moves for shifting the relationship between 'stage' and 'audience', and between different kinds of agency and function.

Typically, a Forum intervention takes the form of an action or statement which says: 'No, I will do/say otherwise'. It's then the job of the Joker to encourage interrogation rather than simple acceptance. The ability to engage in complex 'play' depends on openness, willingness to recognise alternatives, and readiness to negotiate, leading to a consensual 'scripting' of one or more further propositions. Ganguly writes: 'I feel that Theatre of the Oppressed is not only about scripting the play, it also scripts the power within individuals and within the collective' (2010: 120).

Scripting occurs as a response (or 'opposition', as it is characterised above) to the specifics of time and place and situation. In JS's case these are principally things which '[prevent] collective thinking, debate and participatory politics' (121), uppermost among them being caste, gender and religion as they are colonised and manipulated by power structures. Ganguly details ways in which, in rural West Bengal, this is played out in economic and practical terms: healthcare, education and employment are particularly affected by widely differentiated levels of provision according to the make-up of the receiving communities (121–2). In a mainstream Hindu village, there are five teachers per class; in a 'Scheduled Caste' location, one for four classes. Provision follows Party allegiance: 'caste is often used to conceal forms of political and economic discrimination … similar kinds of marginalization and oppression operate under the cover of religion or traditional gender roles' (123). For instance, 'only 12 percent of Muslims complete secondary level education' (124).

In a similar way to Ganguly's discovery of new modes of thinking in response to the material situation in the villages, the methodology of Forum fosters collective thought, deconstruction and scripting in response to the circumstances of daily life. Forum, and the

empowerment it delivers, is thus a strategy to deconstruct the author-
ised narrative promoted by those in power, and to claim a more extensive and active model of democracy, as the title of the book proposes.

> Forum Theatre:
>   animates – problematises – ironises
>   is a process of exchange and dialogue
>   arises from collective input (scripting)
>   validates local cultural resources and intelligencies
>   enlivens and empowers public space

RELATIONSHIP, THE EGO AND THE REVOLUTION IN MIND AND BODY

Ganguly is fond of quoting a story about Mullah Nazruddin. The Mullah
takes a long journey to see his teacher. On arrival he knocks at the door.
A voice from within asks: 'Who is there?' Nazruddin replies 'it is I'.
There is no answer. The scenario is repeated several times. Finally,
Nazruddin changes his response to 'it is you'. The door opens (adapted
from Ganguly 2017: 134; also in 2010: 142–3).

Really meeting anyone or anything in pretty much any situation is
only possible if you are prepared to embrace the unknown, to listen and
be open, to not rush to conclusions or defences of your own intellectual
or social capital. Ganguly sees this as a passing beyond ego, and suggests
that in addition to or commensurate with the 'I/it' perspective, a failure
to do so is a major block to the collective action JS aspires to. He says:
"The biggest obstacle in creating a collective is the "I". Not that the
function of 'expert, leader or director should not exist', but that 'they
are also part of the collective' (2010: 130).

Socialism may aim to create a system which operates 'for the sake of
society in general', but it has never really achieved this goal, because it
'has crucially failed to … acknowledge that aspect of revolution inside
the human being which is not economic in nature' (136). For Ganguly,
the vital ingredient is to recognise that '[t]he relationship of individual
to collective is a simultaneous intellectual and emotional journey. The
experience of that journey is an aesthetics of life' (ibid).

Since Ganguly understands the nature of relationship to be fundamental to this process, JS's work can be seen as a continuous evolution of a practice of relationship. 'A relationship grows out of mutual trust and respect'; and '[i]n Indian tradition the basis of relationship is debate' (137). That relationship moves from respecting, listening to and engaging with the concerns and propositions of participants in Forum, and in workshops, through the deployment of 'mutual gift' or exchange in establishing HRPCs and other community structures, and to the methodologies and principles which govern their operation. In JS's work, social relations have become a 'malleable world of possibility'; that work is a 'resource for strengthening civil society' (Da Costa 2010a: 624) which delivers 'community empowerment through culture' (628).

The sequence Ganguly sets out on p. 137 also reflects this:

> The connection between the spectators as a group and the spectators and the actors develops into a relationship. At this stage the play becomes a collective action where the individual identity of the actors and the spectators merges into one identity.

In Forum Theatre, both the participants and the politics of the situation are subjected to a process involving relationship. The basis of this is establishing connectivity and collectivity, and is presented as:

Actor + Spectator > Joint Social Action + Reflection
= Collective Action (137)

These ongoing processes over time produce complex and fundamental changes of behaviour across a variety of modes and lead to wide-ranging community outcomes ('strategic change': 139), which will be exemplified in the next section.

JS's plays, and the work which frames and underpins them, take its participants on this journey from 'positive conflict' through 'strategic thinking' to 'deliberative action', nurtured by an 'aesthetics of life', which enlivens hope, desire and power. At all stages, this is a 'two-way journey', which 'helps people to experience internal revolution and creates the aspiration for the external one' (142). In Ganguly's thinking here, the self and the collective are mutually supportive; both are 'bigger', more porous, than the defensive or acquisitive position which is often assumed. Ultimately, claims Ganguly, '[a] new model for social inclusion is proposed and tested by Jana Sanskriti's work'.

Sanjoy Ganguly believes that this is because what JS does positions and evaluates human selfhood differently. If you think (live) solely as an individual, egoic entity, you perform in a certain way. You protect your (vulnerable) boundaries. You seek to expand your territory of influence and control. You conceive the world, including the relationship between humans and the other than human, as a set of hierarchies. JS's practice challenges those assumptions because it faces up to the challenges of listening to, recognising and working with the other – as an audience member, an interventionist spect-actor, a member of a co-creative scripting team or a community committee. The self is stretched into a different, porous or permeable (remember Freire?) configuration. I am no longer only 'I'. That of course is also what happens when we act a role, and it is even more evident in Forum when actors have to shift in and out of role continually. I am extended. I become to some degree co-extensive (with my audience, with the spect-actor who replaces me, with the function of the Joker).

In this sense, collective action can be seen as a reconfiguration of self. This extension or redesignation of self is on one hand not just a bit of eastern mystical gobbledegook, and on the other hand not simply an intellectual quibble. If I in some sense also experience myself as you (as Ganguly's Mullah Nasruddin story implies) I am more likely to engage in a politics which is not just about giving myself credit for doing good, or about using you to further my own aspirations to higher status. This has real consequences for real action.

APPLICATION AND EVALUATION

THE QUESTION OF GENDER

In their operational area, JS has focused particularly on gender: '[f]amily violence and family repression due to the existence of patriarchal values are major points of concern of all branch teams' (124). As a result, by 2010, 'women spectators of Jana Sanskriti have formed women's organizations in about 100 villages', and it has a large number of all-women teams (125). As noted in Chapter One, from a situation in which women were discouraged or prohibited from taking any part – even sometimes as spectators – in performance, it has also now been the case for many years that 'when it comes to acting outside the arena, women surely play the most important role in terms of number and leadership' (125–6). Strategies to develop collaboration, training, scripting and organising have thus shifted an entrenched and often unacknowledged set of beliefs and practices.

The importance of learning by being 'spectators of ourselves' is particularly strong in the case of patriarchy: its roots, says Ganguly, 'lie deep within the mind, and this is true for both men and women' (124). Gangly has earlier cited instances of how Forum engagement begins to produce a shift in that mindset for men: JS actors who have begun to ask themselves if the characteristics they portray on stage might still be present in their everyday life, or spect-actors who – however implausibly – seek to humanise an oppressive male character. In the case of women, Ganguly reports that Rainbow of Desire and 'cops in the head' techniques (as for Bakam) have been instrumental in JS workshops in opening up space for them to acknowledge their situation, using the collective agency of the group to support introspection, discover potential responses and script scenarios in which to test them out; thus, far from being only an individual focus, introspection also 'turns out to be a mode of social observation … collective action and introspective action … become complementary' (125).

The changes in social life resulting from shifts in gender relations have been the subject of research projects, as Ganguly notes (126). It's therefore useful here to take a closer look at a couple of studies which have examined aspects of this major contextual reality of JS's practice.

A survey conducted by the Centre for Studies in Social Sciences, Kolkata, the Centre for Training and Research in Public Finance and Policy, Kolkata, and the World Bank discusses long-term and fundamental effects on behaviour in relation to JS's operation within communities. The study, entitled 'Theater of the Oppressed Empowers Women: Evidence from India', examined 99 villages and nearly 4,000 women and their husbands (38 of these villages with JS presence over at least ten years), in order to answer the question: '[c]an an intervention [of this theatre practice] change [a] mindset?' (Hoff et al. 2021: 3). That mindset underlies the statistics that in Africa and Asia, 30% of women have experienced domestic violence and 30% of people believe it is justified for a husband to beat his wife (ibid). The survey team interviewed a male and female respondent (separately but simultaneously) from 3,842 households, 1,744 of which were from villages where JS had been present. No JS personnel were involved and JS had refrained from doing performances for four to five months prior to the survey.

Results indicated that in 'JS villages' there was a reduction of more than 50% of married women who were denied participation in major decisions, and a decrease of over 33% in domestic abuse. Moreover, the effect did not depend on a member of the household having seen a performance (Hoff et al. 2021: 1). The report concludes: 'We find that JS had a large impact on married women's role in household decision making and on their willingness to enforce laws to protect women and women's welfare. JS substantially reduced spousal abuse' (Hoff et al. 2021: 43). ('Decision making' refers to the following domains: major household purchases, visits to relatives by the wife, use of contraception, number of children to bear, children's marriages.)

They conclude that 'JS taught new ways to feel and think about gender roles' (ibid). The report uses a range of statistical measures to substantiate its claims, and in addition to the interviews and structured survey questionnaires, the authors also consulted videoed interventions at Forum sessions. They interpret the perhaps surprising conclusion that it is not necessary for everyone to have seen a performance in order for changes to occur as an example of what they term a 'missing variable' in economics: 'the experience and exposure that create cultural categories and narratives' (43). The way in which Forum and the ongoing cultural shift it engenders operate over a period of time results in 'collective story editing' (8), or the reformulation of dominant narratives about gender roles and relations. They note that in other contexts, 'social change is difficult' and 'dysfunctional norms often persist' (4), but JS's work brings about a collective refashioning of the attitudes and beliefs which underpin those norms.

Hence this study is significant in three respects. Firstly, it *brings to the fore the overarching nature and significance of Jana Sanskriti's approach to questions of gender*, which run through virtually all its work, as issues in the plays, as encounters with incultured belief structures and as nodes of relationship between performers, spectators and communities (let alone in terms of representation and agency in political governance and delivery of key services such as healthcare and education). Secondly, *it provides quantitative measures of the effects of JS's work and triangulates it from the perspective of economics and sociology*. Reductions of over 50% of the number of women who were denied a role in decision-making, and over 30% in respect of spousal violence are in themselves quite significant (JS report that domestic abuse is almost entirely absent from villages where they work, and child marriage has decreased exponentially). Thirdly, the paper also *registers the need to adjust quantitative measurement parameters to acknowledge and assess ways in which shifting cultural practice leads to demonstrable social shifts*. This can be paralleled with Ganguly's claim that material change and political transformation require an understanding and skilled practice of aesthetic process and an art of relationship. Culture is not just an add-on or an uninflected channel of top-down information-delivery: it is part of the weft of interaction and behaviour which composes and fashions people's lives.

Many of these areas are addressed by a second recent evaluation from the perspective of participatory communication. Jhana Brahma, Vinod Paravala and Vasiki Belavati's ethnographic study 'examines Forum Theatre as a form of participatory communication for social change', focusing in particular on how it 'addresses patriarchy, child marriage, domestic violence, and maternal and child health related issues' (Brahma et al. 2019: 1). The article looks at how JS's practice 'subverts the passivity inherent in the communicator–receiver model of the dominant paradigm by activating the critical consciousness of the spectator' (ibid). It posits their use of Forum as a refinement of the concepts of communication, participation and development, all of which have been critiqued in recent times.

The article is based on a qualitative participatory evaluation (February 2018), carried out after one year of a project implemented by JS in the Pathar Pratima Block of South 24 Parganas, 'addressing some critical gender issues through Forum Theatre: early marriage of the girl child, school dropouts and child trafficking prevalent in the project area' (ibid). (In this block, the poverty ratio is over 40 per cent, and there is a female literacy rate of under 40 per cent.) Project methodology included interviews, group discussions and participant observation: with facilitators, teachers, local groups, elected representatives and adolescent girls. Some 90 people were involved, 75% of whom were female.

The study notes that '[JS's] communication approach is clearly bottom-up, radically participatory, community based and led by the oppressed' (ibid: 7); the evaluation found that 'at a microlevel, there is a perception that attitudes and behaviour towards the girl child in the villages have visibly changed' (ibid: 8) – thus confirming findings from Hoff et al. discussed above. Specific examples include: reduced discrimination against girls, reduction of child marriage and willingness to pay dowry, permission for girls to engage in sports and theatre (the Block President claimed that the incidence of child marriage had reduced from 40% to 10%). Older women reported increasing autonomy and development of skills and confidence. Many of these areas involve deep-seated attitudes and change comes slowly, but the JS process facilitates this:

> positive changes in gender relations are not always an outcome of radical and revolutionary acts, but a product of, often invisible and slow, processes of complex negotiations by women to earn their independence and freedom and to be able to participate in the public sphere.
>
> (ibid: 9)

The writers observed a performance:

> in a village called Baddimod, in Dakshin Raypur GP of South 24 Parganas district, where child trafficking was reportedly on the rise, by the Ramnagarabad Theatre team, one of the local Forum Theatre teams of JS. All the performers, except for the 'Joker', were women. Women also played the roles of men in the play.
>
> (ibid: 9–10; see below, Chapter Three for an account of the play)

A lively Forum session followed, mostly focused on alcohol consumption by men, which was seen by the spectators as a major underlying cause of the situation. The session thus highlighted an issue which was in a way unexpected:

> Bandana Bera Biring, one of the actors in this play, explained: 'The focus of the play became alcoholism because that is the reality in their villages'. She suggested that people were quite conscious that the mother is also a victim of strong patriarchy that exists in families and communities and they wanted to bring out that aspect in the play.
>
> (Ibid: 10)

Other interventions raised contextual issues like education, legal resources, government schemes etc.; and pointed to 'the need for exercising collective responsibility of the community toward their neighbours and for showing greater alertness to things that are happening in their neighbourhood, state politics and policies that affect their lives' (ibid: 11), as further possibilities of addressing the situation.

Thus '[t]he play clearly functioned as a trigger for dialogue and incited critical thinking among the villagers' (11). As spect-actors 'came forward to ask some tough questions of the girl's parents, they were actually directing the entire community to reflect and find answers to those questions' (ibid). The article concludes: '[t]his study of JS suggests the strong possibility of changing regressive social norms by harnessing the potentialities of Forum Theatre' (ibid: 12).

It also gives further evidence of the overarching concern of much of JS's work. When Ganguly was awarded an Ibsen Foundation Scholarship in 2017, it was to produce a version of *A Doll's House* which reflected the context of 'patriarchy in West Bengal'.

Sameera Iyengar's 2001 thesis argues that the conception of 'the masses' espoused by progressive political movements 'makes for the creation of a normative individual' who represents them, and because women are associated with the private rather than the public domain, this individual is by default seen to be male and 'women are effectively non-existent' (Iyengar 2001: 94). She identifies JS's behaviour as significantly different, since women became involved in both performance and organisation from an early stage, and as Hoff et al. note, the fallout from this is cumulative. At first, 'women join the organisation with the approval of society'; thus 'society gets used to the fact that women do such work'; and as a further consequence, 'women discuss, analyse and address the problems which they personally face, a move which *must* cause social rumblings …' (Iyengar 2001: 96). Jana Sanskriti's model, however, is not an antagonistic one ('overthrowing one set of people to empower another'), but 'follows a politics which bides its time, moving step by step towards larger goals' (96).

This is significant both as analysis and with reference to tactics. As Kelly Howe points out, patriarchy is 'a set of social relations' which 'plays out within and *composes the very fabric* of … life' (Howe et al. 2021: 130–1; italics in original). Although it manifests in individual actions – and JS plays provide both specific examples and general categories of these – to attack it there is not enough: 'patriarchy is a relational system' (ibid), and any really effective challenge needs to be systemic and sustained. As an 'age-old problem', it cannot be 'solve[d] … on stage' (Ganguly 2017: 94); it needs a long-term strategy. Ganguly identifies key stages in this as 'scripting the play', becoming 'spectators of their own reality', and understanding that patriarchy does not operate 'in isolation from aggressive capitalistic development' and other wider scenarios (2017: 91; 107). 'Forum theatre can lead them to understand that it is not a question of a family, it is not a problem between a man and a woman ... patriarchy is operating in the psyche of the oppressor' (ibid: 94).

In an interview, Poutot asks Ganguly: how does JS deal with 'traditional problems ... such as patriarchy?' (Ganguly 2017: 106). Ganguly begins his answer by problematising the question. He points out that tradition is only one of the factors and influences which make up or enshrine patriarchy, interacting with contemporary political and economic pressures. There are no easy solutions. Systems and values are interdependent.

> So when we are going to perform a play on oppression of women, for example, we're not trying to change a tradition. We are actually trying to find the irrationalities in the modern system ... The whole question of unequal power relations between men and women has always been nourished by the system imposed upon people.
>
> (2017: 108)

Howe concurs:

> Women, LGBTQIA individuals, non-binary individuals and others who suffer at the hands of patriarchy are also frequently its agents, having internalized its power relationships and living them out on the body, even policing themselves with the very norms that have disciplined them.
>
> (Howe et al. 2019: 131)

In this, she echoes Ganguly's comment that 'patriarchy is an ideology and it can be followed by women too' (Ganguly 2017: 92).

Ganguly's response to Poutot adopts the same procedure as that which characterises JS's methodology across the board: recognising and delineating the issue, identifying structural causes, interrogating contextual dimensions and exploring possibilities of response. This kind of holistic thinking and the behaviour it inspires is a means to engage with systemic patriarchy and change societal behaviour. It stands in opposition, as an aesthetics, an ethics and a politics, to the 'quick-fix' and 'soundbite' society which increasingly threatens organic human performance in a whole range of senses.

WORKING WITH GROUPS IN OTHER STATES

In a chapter headed 'Beyond West Bengal: Other Indian Scenarios', Ganguly provides some examples of the contexts, issues, processes and outcomes of JS's collaboration with activist groups elsewhere in India. In discussing these *applications* of the JS methodology, Ganguly reflects on what they bring out in relation to fundamental principles of JS's practice (development of thinking > collective agency > new politics), enabling him to explicate their effects in terms of political action and group behaviour (which also includes aspects of cultural behaviour).

The chapter looks at JS's involvement with:

- Delhi Shramik Sangam, working with migrant labourers in slums
- Savahara Jana Andolan (Maharashtra), working with the Katkari tribal community
- Mallabhum Adivasi Kisan Mukti Sangatham (Orissa), working with the Ho tribal people

The major conditions and issues which the groups were confronted with are:

- migrant labour in the informal sector in cities, its role in the economy, the economic and pragmatic difficulties of workers (travel, schooling, accessibility of work etc.)
- class distinctions
- marginalised rural communities and caste hierarchy
- land ownership and access
- superstition as a weapon of power

These form the key components of oppression. People in these groups have been devalued, disadvantaged and exploited; their track through these situations has been charted in the plays they have created and the processes by which they developed and performed them, leading to outcomes in which collective agency has been enabled to challenge the status quo or the power of dominant interests. Working with Forum process has enabled them to recognise, analyse and articulate their struggle against these factors and to move towards collective agency, and to avoid over-simplifying problems or accepting ready-made 'solutions'. Ganguly says: 'I continue to make conscious efforts through workshops to shift these non-party activist actors ... from the propaganda mode to the interactive mode' (92).

In Delhi, the migrant workforce is 'very useful' but precarious, easily displaced by successive phases of development, often resented by those in more permanent occupations and accommodation, liable to summary eviction (2010: 90). Although caste is not a major factor in marginalisation here, class is; but in response, Ganguly says, 'these uprooted people have been able to build up a unique relationship ... despite having come from various parts of the country' (91). This solidarity is strengthened in the course of developing plays on the issues which affect them and by being members of the (political) organisation which supports the work. One play, *Mera Bharat Mahan* (*My India is Great*), led to the establishment of a non-violent movement which resulted in people being allocated a plot of land by the Delhi Development Authority (91).

The Katkari community suffer caste-based discrimination and exploitation and have repeatedly had to engage in struggles over their rights to water and land. One of their plays dealt with the proposal to create the largest SEZ (Special Economic Zone) in Asia by acquiring 50,000 hectares of land from peasants in Maharashtra (a case similar to that of the protests at Singur and Nandigram in West Bengal referred to in Chapter One). The Forum play created by the group in 2006 highlighted the issue and ultimately resulted in a hunger-strike which gained huge support and led to a revision of the proposal; along the way, community solidarity also thwarted attempts by 'musclemen', paid by a multinational which wanted to profit from the deal, to disrupt the performances (95). The group also, along with the Delhi team, made a play about corruption in the food distribution system, which profoundly affects both communities. In both cases, local politicians were subsequently persuaded to engage with ration dealers, leading to improvements in the system, notably in the case of the Katkari, who, '[f]or the first time ... started getting grain at a cheap, subsidized rate' (93). Thus the play and its outcome was a significant moment in the empowerment of the community, signalling 'the ability of marginal people to progress' intellectually, socially and politically (94). Ganguly is clear that building theatre teams in this way allows the 'complex web of social relations' which govern the lives of these communities to emerge and become available for negotiation (95).

In Orissa, creating a play about malaria, superstition, medicine and power gives evidence that these tribal people, in spite of their degrading designation by higher castes, are quite capable of understanding the underlying structures of their situation. The play shows how political and economic agents use superstition – blaming malaria on a supposed 'witch' – to designate a scapegoat and avoid the responsibility their position should require. Moreover, subsequent discussion reveals that the medical provision the majority of people would actually opt for is largely lacking; demands for this and for improved educational opportunities became central to the organisation's aims (97).

As Ganguly notes in the case of the Delhi group, the plays he prepares through workshops with all these groups are 'a synthesis of their experience, and my shaping up and application' (90–1), and the groups go on to produce further scripts themselves. This interchange of skills and competencies is a mark of participation in the sense he refers to it above; and it signals the way in which theatre process can liberate and deploy those knowledges which are already inherent in the group. Theatre gives the group 'courage and self-confidence to fight in an alternative way' (91); for the Maharashtra team, who mostly comprise women victims of untouchability, their play on the land issue demonstrates the ability to analyse and articulate the root causes of the situation in spite of their exclusion from education and their marginalisation from society (94).

DEVELOPMENT DRAMA

Dia Da Costa's *Development Dramas: Reimagining Rural Political Action in Eastern India* (Da Costa 2009) offers another angle of evaluation. It positions JS's theatre activity as a way of critiquing 'meanings of development, political action and rural futures' (2009: 5). As we saw in Chapter One, the CPM/LFG in West Bengal argued for a policy of industrial investment which effectively closed down alternative views of what development might be. Da Costa argues that JS's Forum practice and its methodology of engagement are a way of resisting this 'dispossession of meaning', and at the same time asserting the value of culture as a means of struggle (19).

Da Costa, who travelled through the villages with JS theatre teams in two districts of West Bengal, South and North 24 Parganas, between 1999 and 2008, exemplifies this by accounts of their plays. *Development* (*Unnayan*) exposes the stitch-up between the communist government and a capitalist multinational enterprise (see Chapter Three for more detail), most tellingly by use of comic irony in dressing the 'Tata' character in the red flag and by portraying Tata as a puppeteer who controls both the Chief Minister and the Industry Minister. The play on illegal alcohol production (*The Bane of Drink*) identifies 'domestic violence and [effects on] liquor consumers' wives' livelihoods as a problem of material and representational inequality' (267). So specific economic and social issues are more tellingly excavated by the dramatic process. Whilst the former play undercuts the monologue of economically driven development, the latter reveals the underlying patriarchy which condones the system and sidelines the distress which impacts women, 'because ... the patriarchal state [only] conceives of materiality through a male optic' (228).

Theatre is a way of doing politics then: Da Costa remarks that her aim is to show what it means to build a struggle around 'means of representation' rather than 'means of production' (269). As in her edited collection of essays on JS (Da Costa 2010b), she emphasises that JS's work juxtaposes real and fictional space as a way of presenting alternative scenarios to those offered by systems of power. For JS, she claims, *alternatives are always available*. Pointing out that capitalism is, among other things, a cultural formation, she notes that it is therefore cultural work that can provide 'a lens into the relationship between processes of meaning-making and the continuing formation of multiple histories of power'(18). A review comments that the book 'convincingly shows how political solidarity and political action grow out of social interactions both on-stage and off-stage'. It depicts 'how rural people – including very poor ones – become actors and script-writers on-stage as well as 'nodes' that generate political activism off-stage' (Kapadia 2012).

Da Costa challenges the usual 'development' wisdom by asking why JS theatre activists who battle against 'the constant normalization of a world of shrinking possibilities and social relations' should be regarded as idealists, 'while those who acquiesce in neoliberal capitalism's normalizations are considered realists?' (2009: 9). She takes this argument for wider dimensions of vision further by arguing that '[s]mall spaces of hope and reimagined political action', such as JS's political theatre, 'can also be significant expressions and struggles against dominant epistemes' (269).

Da Costa's book thus examines the nexus between development politics and the capacity of drama to operate as activism. It also highlights the importance of collective interaction and signals how JS's work engages with a wide spectrum of means of understanding social and political behaviours. In this respect, it corroborates the perceptions registered by the studies on gender and social mores discussed above. It is interesting that these evaluations derive from social studies and development politics, rather than being theatre- or performance-based. They manifest an astute understanding of the methodologies of performance in context, whilst also shifting the idea of performance into a wider domain than that of simply acting on stage.

Da Costa emphasises that affective (emotional) qualities are in fact equally, if not more, pragmatically useful to the confrontation of real-world problems than are ideological tenets. The previous sections on Application and Evaluation above aim to suggest that Ganguly's drive to articulate a broad vision of the self in its relationship to the collective is neither an 'arty' or 'mystical' aberration, nor bourgeois indulgence, but a precise insight into processes of human development in an extended sense, which includes, but is not confined to, the material dimensions of politics and social interchange.

WORKSHOPS AND INTERNATIONAL CONTEXTS

In this chapter, through the writing of Ganguly and others, we've looked at the principles underlying JS's practice, and at applications in India, particularly with reference to issues and plays. This has identified the fundamentals of a working methodology, and shows how what was developed in West Bengal could be applied in other Indian states facing a variety of issues (e.g. urban problems of employment; status and rights of indigenous tribes); thus implying the possibility of the method migrating across cultural, linguistic and societal borders, as well as identifying the key components which underpin its effect. Two aspects which extend the remit further are the training process (what I earlier called a 'longitudinal pedagogy'), and the question of transferability outside the Indian context.

In another section of *Jana Sanskriti, Forum Theatre and Democracy in India*, Ganguly discusses the use of workshops as a pedagogic process and reflects on some distinctions between responses from Indian and western participants. He identifies a 'special feature' of TO as 'tak[ing] the audience through a systematic thought process' (99) and thus sees the workshop activity which moves participants towards scripting plays as an example of this (Chapter Four below describes key exercises which deliver it).

A vital ingredient, which workshops attempt to stimulate, is the capacity to frame and articulate experience *aesthetically*, as metaphor: Ganguly recalls 'people in the village who have no formal education' using song and poetry to 'identify the cause of an effect that they find in their local reality' (98). And he locates the underlying aim of his work as the drive to use these capacities as an act of collective democracy.

So, whether the participants are the 'agricultural workers and small farmers' he normally works with, or the 'social workers, psychiatrists [and] teach[ers]' he encounters in Berlin (98–9), or those attending other workshops in Germany, France, Kyrgyzstan and Bangladesh, the trajectory is similar, even if the responses to particular exercises are very different, because they occur within different sets of circumstances and attitudes. Ganguly reports on using Boal's 'Colombian Hypnosis' exercise with Indian participants in Rajasthan, and Europeans in Germany (Berlin) and France (Manosque). His version 'attempt[s] to make the hypnosis exercise [see Chapter Four for a description; original in Boal 1992: 51ff.] into an "image-reading exercise"' (100); the images are different depending on the culture they emerge from, because 'every exercise in the dramaturgy of Theatre of the Oppressed has its origin in social experiences' (101). He observes that, when reflecting on the images made by pairs working as 'hypnotiser' and 'hypnotised', Indian participants tended to identify situations of concrete oppression: husband/wife, political leader/people etc; or in another exercise making an image to represent what 'theatre' meant to them, they saw objects and actions like 'water tank, bull fight'. Europeans, on the other hand (and urban citizens in India) consistently found it difficult to identify material and factual incident, and instead gave general descriptions and abstract or symbolic interpretations ('struggle, promise, solidarity') (100–2). And when playing the well-known TO 'game of knots' (Boal 1992: 62–3) (linking hands, participants move under and over each other, tying themselves in a knot, and are then asked to attempt to undo it, sometimes with eyes closed), whereas Europeans 'play gently ... try to be calm ... some people even say they enjoyed [it]', in Rajasthan the 'participants were extremely restless, they talked too much, it was chaos' (102–4).

These cultural differences seem similar to Boal's account of how his more 'internally' focused techniques ('Cop-in-the-Head' and 'Rainbow of Desire') arose when he moved from Latin America to France. Ganguly speculates about what they signal about understandings of 'freedom' (or its opposite) and 'hope', and suggests that 'independence interpreted by the system based on consumerism can lead us towards individualism, which is against freedom' (111). 'Freedom', he writes, 'is not only economic independence … it includes the right to an intellectual journey … and access to art' (ibid); above all it derives from the possibility of 'collective relationship' (104). That depends on being able to establish an interfacing of self and other, which as noted above is stimulated by the self-scrutiny inherent in Forum process. The business of creating work jointly and agreeing on roles and responsibilities, which is part of the process of the workshop method, is a preparation for this. So he concludes: 'freedom means relationship, freedom means to feel a part of a collective, freedom means the non-existence of the "I"' (111–12).

Theatre here is a process of seeing oneself in others and others in oneself (what Ganguly calls 'co-directional movement' parallels Freire's 'transitivity of consciousness' referred to earlier). From this emerges a recognition of what is shared and a realisation of the possibility of mutual support in negotiating it.

A lively Forum session brings many spectators into coherence – even if it is the coherence of wanting to debate further, to go on arguing the issue. Ideally, workshops offer the chance to explore these sometimes difficult, but ultimately enriching, collective acts of production. Ganguly here writes about workshops and the performances which arise from them as processes and forms of relationship, as a testing ground for the move towards new thinking and collective action.

For him, such shifts have not only a psychological and political sense, but can also be understood as an ethics and as examples of morality. Morality, he argues, is not solely a private affair: '[e]very morality is a social morality', which has an 'impact … on the individual and the collective' (115). And morality is not just 'good' or 'bad', it is a way of responding actively to a demanding situation: it is performed, not merely explicated. 'Workshopping' then is an ethics and a practice which is consistent with the visions and goals which JS embodies. And although Ganguly is responsible for virtually all of the written reflection on how this occurs, that practice has emerged as a result of the continued input and intellectual engagement of the whole core team and many other actors, spect-actors and activists who make up Jana Sanskriti.

3

PLAYING FOR A CHANGE

Jana Sanskriti plays 1985–2020

OVERVIEW AND KEY FACTORS

Jana Sanskriti's performance work ranges from short Forum plays to new Bengali versions of full-length foreign texts. This is in itself relatively unusual for a TO company, as is the fact that a number of plays have been published in a unique format. This chapter looks at plays from all the categories and:

- examines their focus and their dramaturgy
- places them in the context of the major concerns, political and theatrical, of the company
- asks what acting in/directing/staging them shows about i) making theatre; ii) doing Forum Theatre

A list of JS's plays can be found in the Appendix at the end of the chapter.

The plays in the first part of that list – the majority, ranging over the whole of JS's existence from 1985 to the present – were created with the communities whose lives are impacted by the issues they focus on. In all there are 23 original plays (5 on patriarchy, 18 on other political issues).

The first play, *Gayer Panchali* (*Song of the Village*), is a collection of episodic scenes of village life arising from the early days of JS's presence in the rural community, dealing in particular with the need for men to migrate to the city for part of the year in order to earn enough

DOI: 10.4324/9780429288753-3

to support their families on the land. (They also migrate to other parts of India.)

Although the operation of Party-dominated political power cascaded down to village level also figures here, it is explored much further in the subsequent works, *Sarama*, *The Brick Factory* and *Where We Stand*. (Both Bengali and English titles are given in the list of plays; I will refer to them mainly by the names which JS tend to use most frequently when referring to them.) These plays highlight corrupt practices used by local politicians to hang on to power and access to money, which result in rape and murder. As in *Gayer Panchali*, the impact of these circumstances on the family life of the inhabitants, over and above the general oppression and exploitation of the agricultural workers, is devastating. During the first period of their operation (1985–97) when these plays were created, JS, in combination with other movements, conceived and carried out the enormously demanding 55-day performance and cycle rally (1989): playing *Gayer Panchali* every day on the way to Delhi in order to present a petition and demonstrate in support of guaranteed minimum wages for the agricultural sector. Acting and activism are already deeply entwined in this venture.

To these should be added what is perhaps JS's best-known play, *Shonar Meye* (*Golden Girl*), which depicts key scenes from a woman's life before and during marriage. It is the first play in which JS explicitly addresses the overarching theme of patriarchal attitudes and the behaviours which derive from it, which continues to figure both centrally in some further plays and continuously as a pervasive factor in many others. In addition to being a 'political society', as Da Costa has indicated, West Bengal, in common with much of rural India, also retains strong elements of patriarchal structure. Thus two key themes of JS's awareness of rural life emerge in the early work.

All these plays and several others constructed in a similar way and addressing key issues will be considered in greater detail below.

The scripts of these four plays appear together in a volume entitled *Where We Stand*, first published in 2009 and later republished by JSIRRI (see Chapter One); the book also contains a more discursive piece entitled *Perspective*, which articulates Ganguly's reflections on and stance towards the nature of politics as experienced in the preceding plays. This collection is something of a rarity both in the general domain of Theatre of the Oppressed and in JS's production work. Forum plays are relatively rarely fully scripted and even more rarely published; so these scripts represent archetypes of JS's practice, of types of oppression faced by rural populations, and to a lesser extent of TO as a whole.

The plays which follow those published in *Where We Stand* (from 2001 onwards) chart the extent of JS's involvement in major issues affecting rural life, such as:

- illegal production of alcohol
- inadequate provision of education
- destructive agricultural practice by multinationals
- land-acquisition in the service of industrialised 'development' schemes
- trafficking of women and girls

They arise from community discussion and involvement and are scripted through workshops and repeated engagement, with the final version usually provided by Ganguly. As the core team members became more skilled and worked extensively with their satellite teams, plays have become increasingly, and sometimes entirely, scripted by these teams to address local issues. The list at the end of the chapter refers in the main to plays 'finished' by Ganguly, though always arising in some measure from collaborative input.

The stories of the plays are in many respects the stories of the players. Ganguly often says JS's plays are not imaginary, but real: they undeniably speak of the stuff of real life. At the same time, this is not 'realism'. The plays deploy all the resources of theatrical semiotics to locate and dynamise that reality, so that it inhabits an 'imaginary' dimension which renders it viscerally and evocatively experienceable, whilst at the same time both framing and interrogating it.

We will firstly look at aspects of the plays as a whole, in order to identify characteristics in common; then move to close reading of examples from nine of them to explore further dimensions and understand how they work in performance. This may look like rather a large number, but i) Forum plays are usually short; ii) the range permits us to identify both different elements of the Forum process and different socio-political issues which the plays engage with. Two further initial comments:

1   Playscripts are not the whole story: partly because they are consciously 'incomplete', because their role is to kick-start emotional,

physical and intellectual engagement with and continuation of the confrontation of the issues and problems they foreground. They are deliberate 'acts of provocation and exchange' (Yarrow in Ganguly 2009: 5). Also, as we shall see, in JS's case the 'performance-script' may differ considerably from the written text, and includes a great deal of image work, metaphorical and symbolic devices, action, proxemics and positioning; the published text of four of the plays in *Where We Stand* demonstrates one aspect of how this works by using a large number of diagrams.

2   JS's choices of performance style are also somewhat differently impelled from those of more 'conventional' drama. Da Costa notes that: 'rather than responding to innovations in theatrical conventions, they have seized upon theatrical histories and innovations to respond to a political climate in contemporary India in order to create a space for alternate forms of political representation' (Da Costa in Ganguly 2009: 9). Hence choices to incorporate folk and mythological elements are deliberate strategies to strengthen the critical perspective which is often found in those forms. Form here follows intention; though as the history of JS shows, there is often not much of a time-lag between experiencing the need and finding a way to respond to it as theatre. In the villages, most people couldn't read scripts; this initially very challenging setback precipitated the adoption of a collaborative, workshop-based strategy of co-devising and 'owning' the evolving script throughout its development. Central to this is the use of image theatre and the resourcing of all material from the life-experience of those making the work. Alongside this, dance and folk song was accessible and engaging for the participants; the use of folk forms provided a basis which was formal and demanding but at the same time directly related to their own cultural experience and was fun to do. For examples, see visual clips in the Gallery section on the Jana Sanskriti website (www.janasanskriti.org).

All Jana Sanskriti plays performed by the core team, and the vast majority of those by satellite teams, start with all the actors singing a song and then performing the *kolattam* stick dance.

• The *song* is expressly political: it conveys collective resistance and the desire for other possibilities in life.

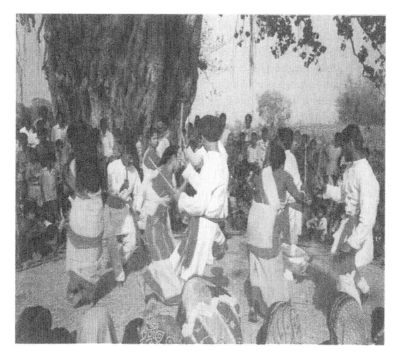

Figure 3.1 Kolattam dance performed at Chandan Keyari, Bokaro, on the border of Purulia (West Bengal) and Jharkand by JS central co-ordinating team (2000).

Photo: Jana Sanskriti

- The energetic *dance* further establishes a dynamic mode which will impel the action and is driven by simple but effective percussion (usually tabla and cymbal).
- Even later adaptation work like *A Doll's House* (*Khelar Ghor* in Ganguly's Bengali translation, meaning 'House of Play/Playhouse'), begins with the actors' *choreographed entrance to chanting*, followed by short single lines spoken by different actors which evoke nodal points and moods of the play to come.
- The *music and movement* – only briefly indicated in the scripted text – focuses and stimulates attention and introduces a theatrical

(aesthetic, metaphorical, but in JS's case resolutely not imaginary in the conventional sense) world.

- For Forum performances in the villages, *lighting* is very basic if used at all, depending on the time of day and available facilities.
- Sometimes suspended *mikes* are used, or sometimes the Joker particularly will use a hand-held mike.
- The *audience* is usually on the same level as the performers, standing or sitting on the ground.

In the early years this 'poor theatre' staging was the only viable option, as most locations lacked regular access to electricity and teams would have to travel quite long distances on foot or by cycle, so very little could be transported. Even now, more sophisticated equipment is expensive and requires time and personnel to set up, so is only used on special occasions such as performances at Muktadhara. At the same time, commercial folk performance in India in the twentieth century did use a range of quite spectacular effects, even if they were sometimes slightly precarious or electrically highly dangerous, in the absence of health and safety regulations. Some of the first JS core team members, who had previously

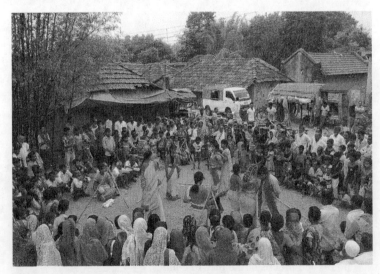

Figure 3.2 JS performance in Purulia, 25 December 2019.

Photo: Jana Sanskriti

worked in local folk performance, were initially dubious about what they regarded as excessively low-key provision. But they soon recognised that such an approach was also part of a strategy which signals that the event is:

- accessible and relevant to everyday realities
- non-hierarchical in its attitude to performers and audience
- deliberately metatheatrical, involving rapid transitions between imaginative immersion and analytical distance
- provocatively political in both narrow and broad senses

Pradeep Sardar writes: 'No light, no stage, a few bamboo sticks to demarcate the stage on the ground, and one lone drum. I felt deeply embarrassed' (Sardar, in Da Costa 2010b: 61). Pradeep Haldar says much the same. But then they note the effect of the performance:

Haldar: 'when we started … everyone was completely silent'; and: 'there was a great discussion after the play'.

(da Costa 2010b: 77)

Sardar: 'after I performed … I knew that there is no greater truth than this'. He goes on to say: 'that's when I understood, there's no stage, no music, no make-up. But in our plays there is soul. This theatre tells people's life stories. That's why I will not be able to give up this kind of theatre'.

(ibid: 63)

This simplicity also applies to what the actors wear. For the most part, they do not adopt complete character *costume*. They may make use of symbolic elements – a scarf, a shirt (particularly if a female actor is playing a male role), a headband or hat; but mostly they work in a basic 'uniform' – men in white kurta and pants with a red sash, women in yellow and red saris (or sometimes variations of this, though usually retaining the clean lines of white and the vibrant colour of red). They signal themselves as actors at work. What turns them into characters is, by and large, the precision and power of their bodies and voices as they materialise those roles; in between scenes or as they change from one character to another, they move with economy and purpose but out of character, or sit at the side of the performance space. Shades here too of Brecht, and for similar reasons. And with links to an older tradition.

Ancient Sankrit drama traditionally starts with a short 'metatheatrical' scene in which the director and a leading performer briefly situate the play to come. The director usually then adopts the function of 'onstage narrator' ('Sutradhar' or 'Bhagawata'): a rather 'Brechtian' role which might appear to prefigure TO's 'Joker'. And in the scripts of Sanskrit plays (e.g. *Shakuntala* by Kalidasa) the dialogue is relatively short and interspersed by frequent descriptions of action or movement. The aim is to produce a highly symbolic atmosphere in which language has a relatively minor part and the meaning of the play's action is conveyed poetically. JS's work thus both follows and departs from this model; its beginnings certainly set out to evoke sensitive and intelligent critique.

JANA SANSKRITI'S INTERACTIVE AND FORUM PLAYS

GAYER PANCHALI (SONG OF THE VILLAGE) (1985)

Gayer Panchali is a series of short encounters between characters which reflect daily realities, for example:

- Sankirtan's decision to leave for Calcutta to find work and his wife Yamuna's sorrow
- Sanatan's need to sell a goat to pay for his mother's funeral rites
- the villagers' hopes that their relatives will return from the city with money for the rest of the year

Two major obstacles present themselves: the economic exploitation of the poor when they do find work; and the manipulation of the system supposed to support them (IRDP: Integrated Rural Development Programme) by local political leaders who siphon off the money.

The play opens with a song, which looks like a standard nationalist paean; but then the chorus asks: 'Can you give us a morsel of rice?' and ironically concludes:

I was born in this country
May I die right here in this country

which is underlined by their statement that 'we are all alive at the mouth of death' (Ganguly 2009: 23–5).

Situation is conveyed by song and movement and by terse but highly charged dialogue. Genres interweave; action is gesture, movement and emotional tone.

The final section of the scene illustrates the workers' plight as the producers of wealth who enjoy none of it. Marxist rhetoric, to be sure, but the facts are that these are the familiar conditions of their everyday lives. The play is 'a critique of ... political society ... in rural Bengal as seen through the eyes of marginalized farmers and agricultural labourers' (Da Costa in Ganguly 2009: 12): politicians use government funds to pay back the money they had to borrow to buy their *panchayat* (village-council-level) seats; workers are aware of this scenario in which politicians simply replace feudal lords of old; 'democracy' wields a stick to retain power. When Da Costa first saw JS's work, she wondered if it was 'melodramatic'. After living with them for some time she perceived that it was not a case of exaggeration. Rather, the brevity and directness of the statements tends to underplay the emotion of the situation: this is *matter-of-fact* stuff:

> We work in the mills, factories, fields, farms ... We are the ones who keep the wheels of civilization turning. Our blood, sweat, and labour makes new creations possible.
>
> (25)

In the first scenes, physicalisation articulates and underlines the textual meanings, using a chorus which operates both vocally and physically. The strained positions of the seated bodies manifest the discomfort of their fragile togetherness; the song on page 28 tells the reality of the IRDP concisely and pointedly:

- the politicians' supporters coalesce into physical form: *'three or four of the actors become chairs in one corner of the stage'* (30)
- any resistance to 'the stick of democracy' subsides literally into the ground: *'the lathis fall from [their] hands ... [a]ll three back off, fall to the floor, and almost merge with the floor'* (36)

The demand for the right to work which closes the first scene is initially undercut by interaction between the chorus of villagers and the 'Interlocutor' (a Sutradhar figure), and then gives way to the capitulation of Sanatan to the exploitative politician Romoni (scene 3). Textual and physical movement traces the same path.

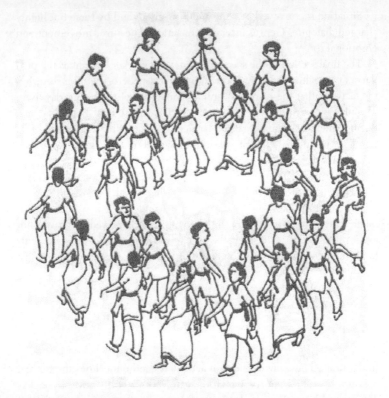

Figure 3.3 Opening of *Gayer Panchali* (*Song of the Village*).

Image: Jana Sanskriti

Figs 3.3 and 3.4 show how this theatre constantly works to redefine its spaces and the relationship and potential of characters and performers within them. JS's performance space is, as already indicated, frequently on the same (ground) level as its (cross-legged sitting) audience. It is marked out by *lathis*, bamboo sticks about two metres long, which are then redeployed throughout the plays in a large number of different ways. The performers not only redesign and reconstruct the 'set' and kinds of action it encloses as they go along (erecting sets of three *lathis* to form a house, or more to form a village; turning one or two into a fence or barrier; using them as signs and weapons of threat and force); they also frequently shift role, from 'chorus' to named character, from human to object or animal (a chair, a goat). Many of these devices of

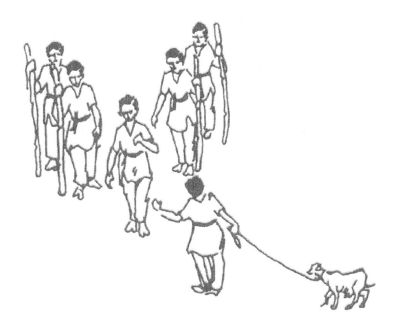

Figure 3.4 *Gayer Panchali*, scene 3.

Image: Jana Sanskriti

physical theatre have become familiar to trainee actors in the west in the last five or six decades (Frantic Assembly, whose work is now synonymous with skilled presentation of subtext through movement in the UK, was founded in 1994, nine years after JS). Here they have extra meaning because the bodies which perform them are in many cases performing the reality of their own lives framed and focused as speaking signs, and because the continuous energy, precision and power which they require to perform is an essential ingredient in the developing recalibration and repositioning of their place in society. When JS performs, the bodies speak of this. Like South African actors under *apartheid*, their play is a site of resistance and an inhabiting of new agency and status.

Scene 6 gives the whole of the Sankirtan story – he leaves for Kolkata, and only the news of his death returns, brought by other villagers. The villagers tellingly conclude: 'The healthcare policy of this government for the poor has ensured the right to death' (47). Sankirtan's story is an echo of that told by Yudhistir Kanaria and recounted by Mohan (2008: 9–10): Yudhistir was a member of the early JS team, who worked in a potato storage unit in Kolkata carrying 60kg bags up a five-storey building by makeshift ladders; he suffered a fall, could not get or afford treatment, and had to return home. He subsequently recovered, but the example illustrates how for many in his position oppression is directly inscribed on the body.

Scene 7 recounts various other ways in which this assessment holds good: a child dies of snake bite, because although snakes live in the village, 'the antidote lives ... in the city' (51); no saline solution in the hospital causes the death of one woman, polio vaccine isn't accessible for another; yet the Chorus ironically intones: 'the country is developing/ Civilization is advancing'.

Scene 8 gives further snapshots of the life of the poor exploited in the city: a man wrongly accused of theft; a woman working as a housemaid raped by the husband in his wife's absence; a young boy violently mistreated by an employer; a worker suffering a fall, like Sankirtan. Scene 9 shows two political parties initially plotting deadly violence against each other and later agreeing to collude to rob peasants of land (similar collusion figures also in the later *Where We Stand*).

The play presents succinct depictions of circumstances and a shrewd assessment of the causes. It *uses dramaturgical means to engage with lived realities*.

Much of the detail is reshaped from the life-experience of JS members: Renuka Das recounts that an accusation of theft was the final straw for her as a young girl working in a middle-class house in Kolkata (Das in Da Costa 2010b: 48–9); the Sankirtan and worker stories derive from Yudhistir Kanaria's experience, outlined above; a similar story about a snake-bite incident affecting their own family is told by Pradeep Sardar (in Da Costa 2010b: 73) and Pradeep Haldar (ibid: 95); violence between the CPM and its main rival the Trinamul Congress (in power after 2011) was frequent, and both sides threatened JS since they feared its ability to speak truth to power – see Ganguly's account of direct attacks on JS actors and an attempt to murder him (Ganguly 2010: 81–3 and 2009: 126).

Dramaturgically, *Gayer Panchali* activates and highlights experience through:

- song, chanting
- swift reshaping of the setting
- sharp verbal exchanges

- the use of masks – as a snake in scene 4, which also calls for considerable physical dexterity; as faceless forces of oppression in scene 8: masks thus function as eloquent signs of realities which are concealed or suppressed
- rhythmic clapping and controlled movement: motion and stillness dynamise and position two Party groups in scene 8; later repetition of the song becomes a kind of keening refrain, as a black cloth is draped over a body

SHONAR MEYE (GOLDEN GIRL) (1991)

Chronologically, *Shonar Meye* belongs with the first batch of plays developed by JS, though the text is not included in the *Where We Stand* collection. It is also probably JS's most-performed play, with many thousands of performances – though *Gayer Panchali* and perhaps *Where We Stand* (the play) would run it fairly close. The striking final image has become

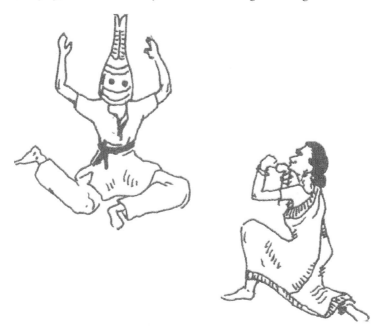

Figure 3.5 Masked figure in *Gayer Panchali*.

Image: Jana Sanskriti

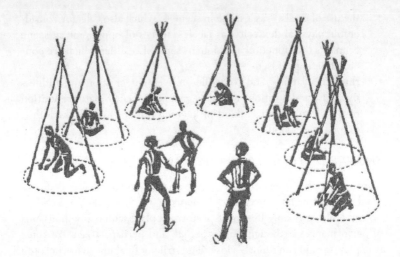

Figure 3.6 Set construction with *lathis*, *Gayer Panchali*.

Image: Jana Sanskriti

iconic as a summary of the style and focus of much of JS's work. The play traces the story of a woman's life before and during marriage, showing:

i) discrimination against the girl-child, Amba – the father angrily prevents her from playing cricket with her brother and then from studying, and orders her to help her mother in the kitchen, whilst her brother is praised for reading

ii) the humiliation of being presented to the prospective bridegroom and father-in-law, who study her physique intently and pass comments: she is reduced to a commodity

iii) the underlying economic oppression exemplified by her father's (illegal but familiar) compliance with demands for dowry – in themselves excessive and threatening to ruin the parents (gold, furniture, a motor-bike and 20,000 rupees ...)

iv) a ritualised marriage ceremony, which ends not in joy but in tears: the father-in-law threatens to stop the wedding as the dowry has not been paid in full

v) how Amba, overworked and mistreated by her in-laws, becomes the butt of aggression after the marriage because some of the dowry remains unpaid; this materialises as physical violence, in which neighbours support the husband and her parents are powerless

vi) her victimisation by the community, who blame her for the situation

The play is framed by an introductory sequence: a song evokes the richness and beauty of the countryside, but the young Amba interrupts this sylvan scene with a cry: 'I want to be free!'

As the dance ends, three women stand facing the audience; three men are just behind them. The women say: 'we want to go out'. The men reply: 'no, women are not allowed to leave the village!'

Thus dance, song, images and sharp dialogue interweave to present the situation: girls can only expect to be married; it is not worth time and money to educate them; roles are gendered and fixed and human systems impact on the bounty of nature.

The trajectory of images runs from joyous play in the forest as a child (other actors represent the forest, make bird and animal noises) through the iconic 'inspection' scene when Amba is statically positioned on a chair and displayed like a puppet, to the final freeze-frame of humiliation and submission in which the forces which condemn her are shown as ropes attached to her waist from each of the other performers encircling her, binding her as she tries desperately and unavailingly to escape. The (live, actor-produced) sound-track includes the forest sounds, a nonsense ditty from the concupiscent father-in-law as he eggs on his rather feeble son, and cutting choric monosyllables ('na' ['no']) in the final image. The scenes are mostly short and pithy (running-time is about 35 minutes and there are about 15 short scenes) and often finish on a stark image of oppression. After a beat, the actors break the image and move briefly into a reprise of the happy dance of the young girl, thus underlining the destruction of her hopes as a constant refrain. This crisp alternation of emotional tone has a powerful effect; it images the situation starkly but refuses to sentimentalise it, thus stimulating both engagement and critique in rapid succession.

A further level of access is provided by a series of symbolic motifs. The composite image of men and women signals the power relationship between genders, which is reinforced a couple of scenes later by a single figure in black. After Amba has played a 'hypnosis' game with her brother (using the Boal exercise) and constructed a linked triangle of their two bodies, the figure appears and declares: 'men and women are not equal!'

After her husband's vicious attack, Amba, prone under a red cloth, has a dream which materialises women's desires of fighting back, in the shape of a mythological goddess in combat with a demon. Two actors turn their backs, don masks and pick up weapons in full view of the audience, then turn and stage a 'pantomime' fight. In Bengal it is Durga or Kali (the latter usually depicted with a highly symbolic garland of men's severed heads); Mudiyettu from South India also features a similar dance/fight between Kali and Darika. Here Indian folk mythology meets Boalian Rainbow of Desire (see Chapter Four below) in a graphic presentation of what in the daytime world is denied to the girl as she passes through the stages of her life (when she says she wants to study, her mother has said: 'I used to have dreams like that too, but nothing came of them'). The dance/fight is not aestheticised in the sense of being concealed; it incarnates the aesthetic power of desire and the intellectual force of exposition in its vital energy and despairing embodied enactment of what women have not been able to say in words.

Following the demand for dowry, three actors in death masks appear to the father. The first represents the sale of land, the second the sale of the house, the third the necessity to borrow money from a loan-shark (Doat 2007: 97). To these speaking images, the powerful moments of freeze-frame throughout need to be added:

- Amba's initial cry for freedom
- the wife on her knees begging the father-in-law not to abandon the marriage
- the final image of the marriage ceremony as Amba bursts into tears
- the husband's raised fist as he prepares to beat Amba
- the concluding image of the ropes as Amba strains in vain to escape

This play often serves as a starter for new satellite teams. It introduces the JS blend of action, music, text and image; it presents a situation which is still all-too-present and recognisable in many locations in which JS operates.

Another play using Bengali music and dance and dealing with a similar topic to *Shonar Meye* is *Giving Away the Girl* by Malini Bhattacharya (2003); and elsewhere in India reports of 'bride-burning' appear frequently in the press and have been extensively documented and investigated in sociological studies: a play by Dina Mehta, *Brides are not for Burning*, came out in 1993. As the evaluations discussed in Chapter Two

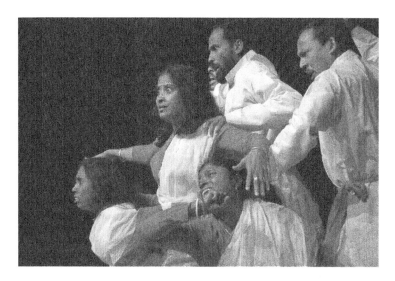

Figure 3.7 JS core team in *Shonar Meye (Golden Girl)*. From left: Renuka Das, Sima Ganguly, Kavita Bera, Satyaranjan Pal, Chittaranjan Pramanik.

Photo: Jana Sanskriti

indicate, JS has had a considerable effect on the span of gender-related attitudes and customs prevalent in the areas in which they operate and recognisable throughout India.

Shonar Meye is visually and rhythmically strong; lively and sometimes darkly comic – especially in the 'inspection' scene, which makes its point strongly through a choreographed routine accompanied by non-sense syllables, as the father-in-law uses his stick to incite scrutiny of Amba's body parts one by one; Poutot astutely notes that here 'language is hollowed out to leave bodies to play out their role to a precise, regular rhythm' (Poutot 2015: 268). This scene, like much of the play, offers a trenchant critique of an immediately recognisable social practice which has severe repercussions on the lives of women throughout India and indeed beyond. Not surprisingly it regularly evokes intense reactions from its spectators, many of whom are prepared to intervene in the Forum. Not all of them are women, although the number and quality of contributions from women right across the age spectrum is striking. Sometimes men start the ball rolling, which is helpful if the audience is new to the process. Sometimes too – as also in other plays, of course – they may try to present themselves in a good light by, for instance, shifting the aggression of the husband or father characters to conciliation or support. JS often do not immediately close down this apparently 'magic' proposition, however suspect it may be. The reason behind this is that by presenting himself (and by implication, male behaviour) in this way, the spect-actor is making a public declaration. The audience may or may not 'believe' him as a viable incarnation of the antagonist; but they will 'read' the statement he is making. Even here they may suspect that he may not stick to his word. But the words have been uttered, and the performative utterance is itself a commitment and an action. That is often a first step to a long process of change.

In his 2010 book, Ganguly recounts two or three instances of (male) spectators and actors recognising aspects of their own behaviour in the character they took on, and the often convoluted process of engaging with it. One of these people was Yudhistir, who, as we have seen above (re. *Gayer Panchali*) was himself the victim of exploitation in his job. In a 'classic' case of cascading oppression downwards, he confessed to Ganguly that he sometimes hit his wife, who not surprisingly was scathing about his claim to be standing up for the oppressed as a member of the JS team. But Ganguly recounts this as a key moment of insight; as with the case of some spect-actors, 'seeing' your own action in a different light starts a revaluation of habit. The 'actor' starts to make the links between the public and private, and without the impetus of the public act this would be less likely to occur.

SARAMA (1992)

Da Costa calls this play 'a scathing critique of the assumption that the party of the poor [she means the CPI(M)] works in the interests of the poor, let alone poor women' (Ganguly 2009: 15).

The play depicts the rape of Sarama, based on a true story of rape by Party hooligans which is then spun as election propaganda by both sides; followed by bribery of the police, muzzling of the Women's Organization in the Party, the absence of effective justice, and Sarama's rejection by her lover after she decides to go through with the pregnancy which results from the rape. The original version then showed Sarama's 'rescue' by the Nirmala Social Service Organisation. (JS core team member Kavita Bera tells of being abandoned by her husband when her child was three days old – in Da Costa 2010b: 106.)

In the play, 'patriarchal rule ... – within the household and within state institutions – helps construct a party-society that collaborates in normalising an ethic and episteme of individual competition and gain' (Da Costa 2010a: 625). This episteme is thus figured/fingered as contributing to relationships of dominance and exploitation, from which Sarama suffers in both public and private domains.

The play's dramaturgy ranges from symbolic choreography (the rapists form an aggressive/defensive triangle vis-à-vis the neighbourhood inhabitants, who later, as chorus, wander around randomly in confusion and fail to find a way to respond) to the use of 'Brechtian' signage (indicating the Women's Organization); it includes the onstage construction of 'set', as *lathis* are used to build Party Headquarters 'to the beat of the drum' (Ganguly 2009: 87), and to create a frame for flashback insertions in scene 5; and switches mode through the use of dream sequences (disembodied voices expressing the incapacity to act, and the absence of 'a place where ... everyone's happiness was possible') and an embryonic 'inner monologue' (ibid: 93) in which Sarama begins to think through her situation.

Short scenes of violent action graphically depict threatening poses by hoodlums, leading to 'rape in broad daylight' (70). The neighbours can only stand still, express their horror, and leave whilst reciting 'Motherland, you know it all and yet you are mute': a despairing call to find a way to move beyond victimhood. But against the background of

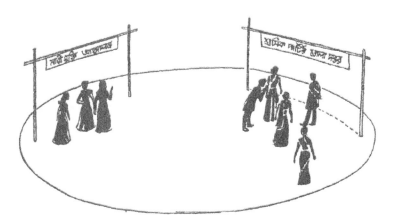

Figure 3.8 Set construction with *lathis, Sarama.*

Image: Jana Sanskriti

Party activity for the men, which is shown to consist mainly of bribery, gambling, schemes to produce illegal alcohol, complicity with corrupt police etc., the following scenes of longer passages of discussion are inconclusive: middle-class women can only play out another kind of deception and cover-up. The women debate what to do and identify patriarchy as an overarching structure, but are effectively sidelined by their own vulnerability to taunts of 'city-derived' feminism and to the overriding claim that the interests of the Party come first, and in the interest of 'the revolution', the incident must be hushed up. Only one woman, Sutapa, speaks with the force and clarity which challenges that power: 'There's no democracy at home, [so] how on earth can there be democracy in society?' (89).

She prefigures Sarama herself, who manages to find a powerful and articulate anger in the court scene, prompting her lawyer to challenge police and legal procedures which have failed to construct an adequate case. In her subsequent confrontation with her lover Adheer, Sarama sees through his protestations of being wronged and ultimately takes off the ring he gave her and throws it at his feet. Although in both these situations she is still violated and as a consequence deeply upset, she begins to find a way to respond. This drive is carried forward into the dream sequence, which manifests her desire to move through her experiences; although as the dream ends she *'seems so tired and her head leans over with fatigue'*, as she says: 'Why can't I see anything? Why is everything so hazy?' (103). The chorus surround her and the Sutradhar starts to narrate how her life turned out subsequently.

Thus performative strategies sustain and extend the insights in the script. However the first version of the play optimistically concluded with Sarama being supported by the Nirmala Organisation to find a new life. In an early performance, this moment precipitated a significant shift resulting from a moment of recognition. After the performance the actors were approached by a group of tribal women who worked in the mines cutting stones, and who had direct experience of the central situation depicted in the play on a regular basis. Ganguly writes that when challenged by a woman called Phulmoni (also spelt Phulmani in places), he and the company were 'speechless'. She asks: 'At [the contractor's] will, we have to visit him alone in his home. Otherwise we lose our jobs. What do you say, shall we leave our jobs? What shall we eat without work? How will we run things, you tell me, mister!' (Ganguly 2009: 66), questioning the possibility of a happy outcome or 'empowerment' in a real-life situation where sex is demanded in return for keeping the job which is the only household income.

From this comes the realisation that 'the question of any social problem cannot be solved by actors and director alone [or indeed by good intentions]. We need to give space to the viewpoint of spectators' (Ganguly 2009: 66). Forum emerges from this; the final scene of the 1992 text was amended to set this up by extending the debate between Sutradhar and actors, and issuing a direct invitation to the audience to engage with the concluding situation and suggest alternative outcomes. (A further consequence of this was an increased desire on JS's part to collaborate with other movements and activist groups – see Chapter One above).

Note that these two 'pre-Forum' plays are the longest of the published scripts, though they are only about 40–50 pages. Forum plays generally are shorter; in both cases the aim is to raise intellectual and political issues as vividly as possible.

THE BRICK FACTORY (ITHBHATA) (1992)

The post-performance encounter after *Sarama* leads on to the *The Brick Factory* (*Ithbhata*). This play exposes the realities of Phulmani's workplace 'and the relations of power that tie her to her work' (Da Costa in Ganguly 2009: 16). The play emerged from work with indigenous Santal and Ho communities in West Bengal and Orissa. The opening song (ibid: 111) establishes a work rhythm for the community, from waking up to leaving for the day's labour; the *lathi* houses back the open space of the stage in which that work is presented as sequences of action (as also in later plays like *Shonar Meye* and *Village Dream*, distinguished by gender, though here both men and women are engaged in different facets of the brick-making process). The 'overseeing' of the work (with prurient undertones in respect of the gaze targeting the women) by the factory owner is also immediately established visually and spatially.

A second song charts the passing of the hours in seven lines (112): Bengalis are perhaps even more given to song – often of a lyrical and slightly melancholic tonality (think perhaps of the music in Satyajit Ray's films) – than other Indians, though everywhere in India and in most Indian performance genres, music is ubiquitous. It resonates both with the regional sensibility and with 'universals' of human experience.

In scene 2, discussion of the payment situation reveals both gender discrimination and exploitation, and the boss's duplicity. Firstly he attempts to divide and rule by appealing to the men's desire to retain an advantage; then he promises but subsequently fails to pay additionally for overtime. Families bear the brunt of this treatment; Phulmoni and her husband row and he storms out; the boss arrives and threatens the sack if he doesn't get sex; the husband returns and witnesses the ensuing violation (120). The whole sequence of description, discussion, events and crisis occurs in ten pages of text; dialogue and action is sharp and succinct, in addition to the role of music noted above. The last scene depicts the trial of Phulmoni (and subsequently her husband) before the village leaders headed by the *morol* (moral leader): the outcome is unjust and violent, encapsulated in the final static images of the play.

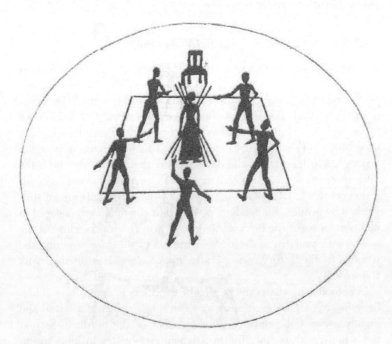

Figure 3.9 Final image from *The Brick Factory*.

Image: Jana Sanskriti

The concluding lines are:

FIRST PERSON: Hunger caused Phulmoni to go to work in the city. Taking advantage of her poverty, the owner forced himself on her. Phulmoni was judged guilty.

SECOND PERSON: But actually the owner is the guilty one. Who will punish him? (123)

In addition to the challenge projected at the end, there are a number of significant moments – several of which are indicated above – which can give rise to potential interventions. However, the problem is pretty intractable. What appears bleak both in material terms and from the point of view of well-meaning intervention is that the structures in which Phulmoni is caught up leave virtually no room for hope: Ganguly says: 'There is no solution to her problem' (Ganguly 2009: 17).

But in spite of this, the play signals an 'engagement with Forum Theatre in much more complex terms' (Da Costa in Ganguly 2009: 17). Theatre is seen as 'not just a tool for instrumental intervention to mobilize around a relevant and topical issue ... nor ...a safe space for political action in times of repression and violence' (ibid). Instead, it has to find a way of negotiating both dead-ends and magic solutions, as well as 'conservative norms which stand in for solutions' [e.g. putting the blame on the victim] (ibid). If it looks as though the protagonist's position at the end is inescapable, it is incumbent on the spectators, with the Joker's assistance, to explore if there is any possibility of shifting the focus from 'solution' to 'causes'; and part of the learning here is to trust that, even in an apparently bleak situation, the audience has the capacity and the desire to entertain that challenge.

AMRA JEKHANE DARIYE (WHERE WE STAND) (1993)

Amra Jekhane Dariye manifests 'disaffection with trade union politics' and the exposure of 'corruption and self-interest' (Da Costa 2007: 295); and commits to a politics which aims to 'find our limit' (296); better, perhaps, to find a way to move beyond it.

The play – a 'heady mix of humour, satire, empathy, melodrama, and analytical commentary' (Da Costa in Ganguly 2009: 14), shows the 'unholy nexus' between trade union leaders, businessmen and politicians, and the way in which people are rendered gullible or confused and/or reduced to 'vote banks'. Ganguly explains that '[t]he unholy nexus between trade union leaders and industrialists ... was known to me', as well as the fact that 'political parties control trade unions, not the workers' (ibid: 126). The play has recently been revived, suggesting that it can still be seen as appropriate in current (2021) times, with some adjustments (the rape scene has been cut and the Party names have been changed – in the original they are, amusingly, the Red Party, the Original Red Party, the Only Red Party and the Most Original Red Party). The basic political scenario still holds good, even if the major parties contesting for votes have different names (but many of the same personnel) as those alluded to previously.

This is a very tight play, only 23 pages in length. It exposes the inter-party 'war over capturing pockets of local power', which characterised relations between political parties in West Bengal for long periods during the rule of the LFG. Succinct depictions of the situation and way it affects ordinary people are delivered through sparse dialogue and graphic action, underpinned by drumming and strong visual images.

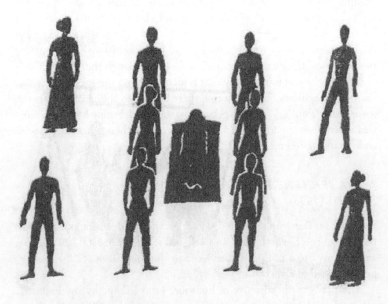

Figure 3.10 Initial image, *Where We Stand*.

Image: Jana Sanskriti

The action moves from the discovery of the dead body of a worker to the corpse's revelation of how he was murdered, followed by an account of the circumstances in which this act arose, and finishing with a series of empty promises from politicians who overpower all resistance.

In scene 1, the workers' initial positivity ('we found a direction to walk towards') is translated into an optimistic pyramid of bodies; but it breaks up, and they walk round the stage in a more uncertain fashion, recalling moments of Communism's chequered history, from the 1917 Russian Revolution to the fall of Soviet Russia in 1989. As these brief statements end, a song leads into the creation of a static formation with the dead body at the centre.

The trade union leader and MP, Tarit, lauds Bikas's sacrifice but stops short of promising any action; in the next part of the scene he accepts a bribe from jute mill owner Manganlal (who had Bikas killed as a potential trouble-maker). Somewhat like a Shakespearean ghost revealing the truth of their murder (e.g. in *Hamlet*, *Richard III*), Bikas rises to his feet and speaks, whilst Manganlal believes he is dreaming. Tarit advises Bikas to go back to being dead, but his account stirs his fellow workers to accuse Tarit of lacking any conscience, as they speak and move rhythmically, and the scene concludes with Bikas standing on a stool holding a red flag as the chorus sings. Throughout this sequence, movement and physical position delineate the dynamics of the scene.

The next four scenes present different aspects of the context of the murder of Bikas and the repression and manipulation of the workers.

The network of conspiracy and control extends to the police – cardboard shields with hats and *lathis* form a wall which conceals their vicious tactic of rape as an oppressive weapon – and Party leaders discuss how to divide up what they regard as vote-fodder before manoeuvring the workers/voters abjectly around the stage like goats.

The final scene is tightly structured and choreographed through movement and action, interspersed with brief text from the leaders. The sequence is:

  i) the four Parties fight over who will control the 'state' (represented by a chair)
 ii) the chorus of hungry people ask for basic food
iii) the leaders listen, look at each other, laugh at the people's request, fight, fall still
 iv) the chorus ask for freedom
  v) repeat of iii) but two parties collaborate against the others

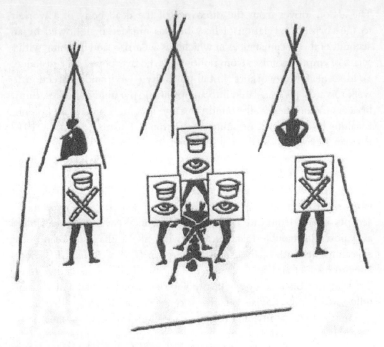

Figure 3.11 Police station, *Where We Stand.*

Image: Jana Sanskriti

vi) chorus approach chair and ask for work

vii) leaders listen, look at each other, move to four corners; call the people with promises

viii) to a drum beat, the people go to one or other of the leaders; they keep running from one to another

ix) all stand still; leaders observe

x) chorus ask for life, healthcare, food, work etc.

xi) the Prime Minister and two other ministers enter and announce a special programme for poverty alleviation. The ministers go to the chorus and attach a rope to the wrist of each chorus member, one by one. They bring the other end of each rope to the PM

xii) repeat announcements by PM and ministers: allowance for widows, reservations for women for jobs, meals for children. At each announcement the chorus, kneeling, bend their heads further as the ropes tighten

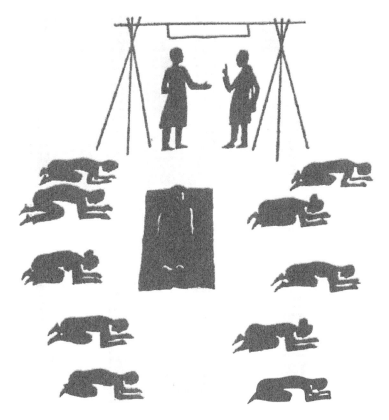

Figure 3.12 *Where We Stand*: Manganlal and Tarit negotiate as the workers mourn the death of Bikas.

Image: Jana Sanskriti

In these plays we have seen the basics of JS's developing dramaturgy, in the ways in which they use bodies, space, rhythms, masks and other elements to activate and physicalise encounters and situations. As their awareness of Forum grows, they are also increasingly concerned to:

- identify and animate (problems, conflicts)
- expose (corruption, hypocrisy, incultured behaviours)
- affect (via shock, sympathy, anger, comedy)

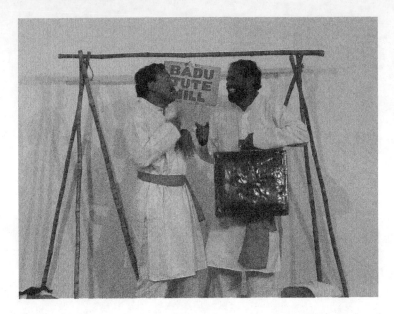

Figure 3.13 Chittaranjan Pramanik and Satyaranjan Pal as Manganlal and Tarit in *Where We Stand*.

Photo: Jana Sanskriti

All the plays operate an interweaving of image and text. They also juxta-pose action and stasis: at the end of many scenes, action is frozen at a point of crisis as an image composed from many bodies, before dissolving into movement or dance and shifting to the next phase of action. The diagrams and images in the text give a sense of how this looks on the stage. What this frequent framing particularly incites is a focused reflection on key moments, leading to a structural analysis of what has caused this situation.

The material arises from the real-life experience of the performers and has an immediacy and authenticity in consequence; shaping it – the work of 'scripting' in workshops and crafting it further as a perfor-mance text in rehearsal – needs an alertness from actors and director so that the situation 'speaks' to the audience and, crucially, invites them to enter into a further dimension of 'work' on it.

It's worth looking back at the accounts above and identifying how bodies, text and action function to present striking moments, iden-tify critical junctures and open space for intervention. Forum needs

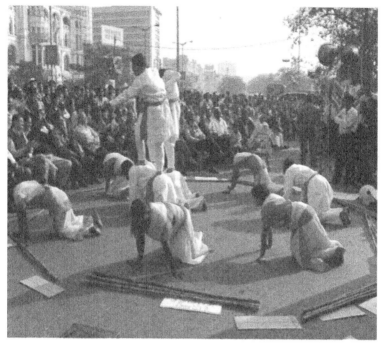

Figure 3.14 *Where We Stand*: party leaders ride on voters' backs.

Photo: Jana Sanskriti

performers who can take on this combination of the 'real', the 'physical' and the 'strange', and mould it into an invitation to the audience to see, think and act. Chapter Four will explore further how training can move towards this.

PERSPECTIVE (DRISHTIKON) (2007)

This play, which is also printed in *Where We Stand*, is more a kind of Platonic dialogue than a performable play. It has only been produced on a few occasions as a stimulus to 'in-house' debates on the key issues it discusses. In a sense the play represents Ganguly's 'manifesto'. The progression which occurs in it is from the closed-minded violence and fundamentalism of Party doctrine to a developing recognition of 'Ranjan consciousness', which includes many strands of what JS has come to articulate. But its form is that of public debate rather than embodied struggle and dramatic action. As it moves towards its conclusion it tends also to become increasingly didactic, though the final image is – perhaps unconsciously – somewhat ambiguous.

Prior to Ranjan's first entry, the 'people' ironically describe themselves as they believe the Party views them: 'we are brainless, without intellect' (153). The Party Leader agrees, claiming that '[f]or the revolutionary transformation of society, this complete theory and submission is necessary' (154). Ranjan on the other hand convinces the people that the Party leaders wear many masks and that ordinary folk have within them the power to change things themselves. A Tagore poem celebrates this vision as people sing 'We are messengers of new life ... /We break the chains of constraint' (160).

The Party Leader asks why they are 'singing those terrible songs'; Ranjan challenges the Party line, engaging in debate and exposing the inconsistencies of its position. The debate is convoluted and often confusingly hair-splitting, though not unconsciously so: a Party representative declares himself confused, which is presumably intended to show the usual nature of this kind of debate; here, it shifts rapidly across political theory, the history of Communism, graft and bribery as political tactics, and so on, demonstrating in its complex convolutions and superficial slickness the way in which leaders both intellectual and organisational may employ these kind of strategies to confuse their listeners deliberately. As the play goes on, some of the Party characters begin to waver and the number of Ranjan characters increases: a 'multiplication' which signals that they are beginning to see the light.

Extrapolating the key points from the argument, 'Ranjan consciousness' implies the following:

- refusal of absolute submission to the Party line
- exposure of the power-seeking of control politics
- ironising, undercutting and challenging standard Party doctrine
- exposing hypocritical claims to champion 'the people'
- identifying intellect, desire and agency in the people
- motivating others to discover those qualities in themselves
- stimulating solidarity and mutual support in consequence

Thus the stages it moves through are: resistance, analysis, dialectics, exposition, encouragement and solidarity.

At the end of the play, all characters join together in 'push[ing a] stone with collective strength' (177); they sing a song whose words are from a Tagore poem:

> In the waterfall of light wash it over
> The hidden and dusty place within you, wash it over
> The person within me who is encumbered by slumber ...

(178)

Ganguly positions the play as a moment of reflection upon his preoccupations rather than as a performance. The fact that there are no diagrams underlines this. As this play shows, he is critical of many of his own tendencies as a thinker and a writer, and not afraid to expose them. It is in this light that the play can be seen, standing as it does at the junction between action and reflection which is such an integral part of JS's process. As we shall see, an element of metatheatrical critique occurs in other JS plays as well. Ganguly says that the play emerged very much from his own reflection on doing politics as theatre and understanding it in the light of earlier Bengali thinkers like Vivekenanda, for whom the 'spiritual' is essentially a process of relationship within and beyond the 'self' and education is a 'realisation of the perfection inherent in [human beings]' (Ganguly 2010: 38–9). Since a key part of that 'perfection' is the potential for rational thought, the play can also be seen as a mark of the continuous self-critique at the heart of JS's enterprise. It is not only a question of interrogating what the plays address but also of asking why, and if so how, plays can do the job.

DEVELOPMENT (UNNAYAN) (2008)

Da Costa places JS's work in the context of 'development': '[e]ach moment of Jana Sanskriti's political action is testimony to struggles in contemporary constructions of development, and battles against alienation' (Da Costa 2007: 308). In the first decade of the twenty-first century, the CPM in West Bengal attempted to promote industry in the state in order to raise its productivity, create jobs and thus, they claimed, to be able to benefit everyone, including the rural poor. Using a model employed elsewhere in India, the creation of Special Economic Zones (SEZs), they proposed leasing some 1,000 acres of agricultural land to the conglomerate Tata for a factory to build a 'people's car' which would retail at much below other models. According to the CPM, 'capital insertion alone resolves West Bengal's agrarian impasse' (ibid) and was presented as a way to prevent the scenario of widespread suicides of farmers occurring in other Indian states, for example Maharashtra, where there were 12,000 between 2015 and 2018. This scenario also relates to agricultural and social policy, and has been addressed by JS's play about Monsanto (*New Agriculture* – see below) and plays and activist projects by their associated group Savahara Janandolan in Maharashtra, which works with tribal people in the district of Raigabh.

However, Satyaranjan Pal of the JS core team 'questions [this] consensus' between government and private capital and asks '[i]s this the only model of industrialisation available?' (da Costa 2007: 307: Pal is referred to in this article as 'Mahesh'). JS's work of course aims to open up 'difficult' questions of this sort, and the play 'show[s] a government that had "previously shown us the path" ... making a "naked" transition by donating land to big capitalists like Tata. The chief minister becomes an object of ridicule as he offers Tata any amount of land, electricity and water' (Da Costa 2007: 310).

The minister cannot find his 'decent attire' because he has sold the red flag to Tata, who happily loan it back when the minister has to face farmers at public meetings, and are 'pleased to be participating in a "new history for Bengal ... which let[s] the people of the world see how Communists love capitalists"' (Da Costa 2010a: 630).

The play is also not without difficulty for JS, as it 'happens to be a protest against the very corporation that funds [some of the activities of] JS' (ibid). And the play also shows how JS use Forum as a mode of critique not only of the issues focused on, but also of its own practice of making theatre: the play opens by raising the question: 'Performing a play? Two days after the land is gone, there's no telling what I will be able to eat, and they are performing a play here?!' (Da Costa 2010a: 630). Aesthetic, ethical and political questions thus underpin the play, which 'risks' a great deal. JS engaged in a conversation with Tata, and although the latter did not renew funding for their work at that time, they have contributed some support on subsequent occasions.

JS's production played a leading role throughout this landmark action over the proposed car-plant at Singur, which was also highly charged politically. JS was in a position right from the start to put forward a trenchant but balanced critique of the different political and community perspectives at stake, because it had been adamant about remaining politically neutral and not accepting funding from any political party. The mainstream theatre scene in Kolkata found this more difficult. Kolkata has long prided itself on its intellectual and artistic prowess, and in no small measure this is connected to the presence of left-leaning thinkers. Links between the ruling Party (CPM) and leading theatre groups were not necessarily formal, but none the less tenuous; so in spite of a long history of 'street theatre' in Bengal, the 'tradition of protest movements ... [was] totally co-opted into uncritical support for the ruling Left' (Biswas & Banerjee 1997: 36). It was not until the degree of antagonism to the Tata proposal became clear that some of these groups felt able to get on board. Some of their leading figures have subsequently aligned themselves with the Trinamul Congress, which was able to capitalise on this key moment in its march to power in West Bengal.

NEW AGRICULTURE (NATUN CHASH) (2007)

This play deals with the monopoly acquired under a government-deal by Monsanto, which locks farmers into using not just their seed varieties but also pesticides and fertiliser. Like the misnamed 'green revolution' years earlier (1960s and 1970s in the states of Punjab, Haryana and Uttar Pradesh), the products initially deliver increased yields, but as time goes on the soil becomes increasingly degraded. Much of India's Punjab state suffered from the effects this kind of policy and degenerated from being the major wheat-provider of India to having large areas of near-desertification. Farmer suicides have also been extensively linked to this scenario in several states in India (see Ganguly 2010: 139; and Da Costa 2010a: 309).

Indian environmentalist Vandana Shiva calls this practice a second Green Revolution. Whereas the first was mostly funded by the Indian government, this version, she says, is driven by private (and foreign) interest – notably multinationals like Monsanto – which may result in foreign ownership of much of India's farmland. Excessive and inappropriate use of fertilisers and pesticides pollutes waterways and kills beneficial insects and wild life; it has caused over-use of soil and rapidly depleted its nutrients.

A film by Anshul Sharma entitled *Mitti – Back to the Roots* deals with farming in India. The young woman protagonist 'learns ... that a vicious cycle pushes high-yielding or genetically-modified seeds to farmers, forces them to invest in hazardous chemical fertilizers and pesticides, to take loans at high interest rates and struggle with drought and unscrupulous traders'. The film depicts suicides and an entire debt-trapped village being put up for sale. There is no government regulation 'because politicians are complicit with the big transnational companies' that sell the seeds and fertilisers (Chaudhuri 2018: 17).

JS's play addresses this scenario, whilst also serving to inform farmers more fully about the factors involved. In order to ensure factual accuracy about the biochemistry, JS arranged workshops with scientists and agriculturalists during the construction of the play. JS was also concurrently developing organic farming practices on some land it owns near Digambapur, and continues to support eco-friendly farming practices in the region.

These two plays, whilst remaining fundamentally Forum events which generate dialogue about causes, effects and appropriate subsequent action, indicate a further dimension of JS's approach, in that they are a direct response to current and very visible situations, and require intensive research to ensure accuracy in presenting different perspectives on the issue. The preparation this involves is a vital part of the actor's job in Forum. For an intervention to engage effectively with the complexities of the situation, actors – chiefly those in the role of antagonists or oppressors, but also 'bystanders' or those with other potential interest or stakes, emotional or financial, in the situation – need to be able to articulate a convincing case for their position. That case has to be 'improvised' in response to a spect-actor/protagonist's new proposals, but it needs to be grounded in plausible detail. These crucial elements of JS's performances are not scripted a-priori, and chiefly exist in the actors' memories. The most frequent interventions are however recorded in note form by the team after the performance, and are stored in Bengali files held at Girish Bhavan.

The following play was developed with support from educational and law-enforcement authorities, aiming additionally to develop provision in communities (e.g. 'watch committees') to monitor the situation and take action on an ongoing basis.

BANDONA THEKE BINDIA [A PLAY ABOUT TRAFFICKING] (2012)

A performance of this play presented by an all-women team is referred to in Chapter Two.

> The protagonist of the play [is] a young girl, daughter of an alcoholic rickshaw puller and a mother who works in people's homes as a maid. The drunk father wastes away all his income in drinking. The family is struggling to send the girl to school and barely able to afford her books and other essentials. Two unscrupulous traffickers from a neighbouring state tempt one of the women in the village with a job offer for her son and in exchange ask her to find a young woman for a 'suitable job' in their state. The woman then goes to the rickshaw puller's wife and, taking advantage of the family's poverty, she and the two traffickers persuade her to send her young daughter for 'work' outside the state. The girl ends up in a brothel with a 'madam' who seems to be getting a regular supply of sex workers through trafficking.
>
> (Brahma et al. 2019: 9–10)

As with other plays, the depictions of what happens to the protagonist are terse and graphic, materialised as stark images and brisk shifts between scenarios. The female performers are powerful and unsentimental in their rendering of the web of oppression and the complicity of both male and female agents in the process. The resultant Forum identifies a complex structure of interlocking factors which lead to the girl's plight. In consequence, it feeds into the ongoing collaboration between members of the communities affected, the police, schools and other agencies, in line with the development of collective responsibility which is often found where JS has worked. It's noticeable that at JS performances, local government representatives – and sometimes MLAs (Members of the [State] Legislative Assembly) – chief police officers, head teachers and other dignitaries make themselves visible, quite often delivering a speech as part of the introductory proceedings. There's an element of promotion and/or justification here, of course; but their presence and endorsement nonetheless represent a public commitment, rather like some of the interventions of men in Forum sessions discussed above. That public statement does not go unnoticed: it has repercussions. 'Public space' is also a locus where action speaks.

TRANSLATIONS AND ADAPTATIONS: THREE RECENT PLAYS

In recent years Jana Sanskriti has produced several translated and adapted versions of published plays from other countries. In each case, the play chosen illustrates aspects of social and interpersonal life which

are recognisable in the contexts in which JS works, although they originate from other times and places. The intentions behind this are:

- to extend the challenge to JS's audiences of identifying central
  issues and analysing the structures of oppression behind them
- to challenge the performers to negotiate different theatrical styles
- to establish a claim for JS's work in more 'mainstream' circles
- to locate that work within a wider cultural, geographical and historical ambit

A VILLAGE DREAM (2011)

The first of these, performed between 2011 and 2015 in several locations, both in Kolkata and in the rural areas, was an Ethiopian play, *A
Village Dream*, by Mesgun Zerai (translated by Sanjoy Ganguly, directed
by Sanjoy Ganguly and Ralph Yarrow).

The play is set 'somewhere in Africa – mountains in the background'.
Opening scenes in the village show the women engaged in back-breaking
labour whilst the men lie about, play cards, or – in a transposition to
the Indian context – watch test cricket on the tv: India versus Paki-
stan. But later the women devise a scheme to open the men's eyes; that
night, they all leave secretly and go into the mountains. The men cannot
believe their eyes when they wake up and find no one to cook the food
and bring in the water, but at length, after much arguing, start to do it
themselves, rather badly. The next night one newly-married girl breaks
the pact and returns to see her husband; as she leaves, the men spot
where she is going and follow the trail of seeds she laid down to guide
her back up the mountain. When they get there, they find the women
ready for them, since on her return they collectively dream of what will
occur (the women are both intuitively sharp and down-to-earth; the
men tend towards childlike pathos and incompetence …); the women
have a proposal which will only see them return if the men take on more
responsibilities. This conclusion suggests that the play itself is in the
African Theatre for Development mould of advancing a solution and a
moral lesson. JS however viewed it as a useful parallel to some of the situations depicted in their own work, and felt it would make an amusing
and instructive comparison, which they underlined by developing the
'folk' nature of the performance, gently ironising the final resolution
and scrutinising some key moments through the use of Forum, whilst

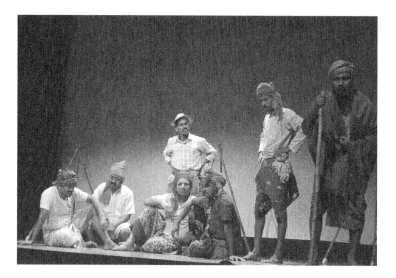

Figure 3.15 *A Village Dream*: the men wonder how to cope.

Photo: Jana Sanskriti

at the same time both validating the desire to achieve consensus and questioning the apparent relative ease of its attainment.

The play offered an opportunity to showcase some of JS's performative strengths and to develop other skills. Physical action neatly and humorously sculpted similarities between rural life in India and Africa (huts made, as usual in JS plays, from *lathis*); and increasing pace when performing repetitive tasks was used to chart the women's daily burden; both this and the scene-shifting dance were precisely choreographed and rhythmicised, and further emphasised by choral singing by all actors, in and out of role (in another example of the performative engagement of people at all levels of the extended JS operation, extra instruction for this was provided by a teacher, a JS associate, who travelled 70km on the train to do this and then went back the same night). Lighting, more elaborate than the usual format – the first performance took place in the ICCR (Indian Council for Cultural Relations) fully equipped auditorium in Kolkata – was also extended to include shadow-play for the young lovers' scene, and projections for the journey up the mountain, during which the women also carried lit candles; costume was more descriptive and included distinctive notes of tribal dress; the men's inept performance of household tasks became a comedy routine, contrasting tellingly with the punitive pace which the women had earlier had to achieve. Journeys up and down the mountain were achieved by descriptive mime.

The live soundscape, evocatively created by the actors on and off-stage, comprised morning, evening and night atmospherics of birds, animals, crickets etc.; wind, rain and the swish of an eagle's wings (part of the dream-knowledge). Although the conclusion presents something of a 'magic solution', the play offered useful opportunities for Forum exploration and recognition of transcultural parallels; in addition, it both underlined existing capacities and opened up new spaces for JS's thinking about performative aesthetics and the status of their work.

THE GOOD PERSON OF SZECHWAN (2016)

The second venture was a version of Bertolt Brecht's The Good Person of Szechwan. This is a play which deliberately poses a largely irresolvable conundrum (how to be 'good' in social terms in a world ruled by acquisitiveness and exploitation). Through it, JS is concerned to ask audiences – precisely, rural audiences – to take up the intellectual challenge of addressing what is also a highly pertinent concern in real life. As we have seen, JS's constituency is encompassed by many varieties of concupiscence, hypocrisy, manipulation, dodgy dealing, and direct threat: all of which behaviours are faced by Brecht's female protagonist Shen Te, who has to call up a hardline male 'cousin', Shui Ta, to rescue her from the exploitation which otherwise threatens to leave her incapable of fufilling her philanthropic tendencies. The point is that collectivist behaviour, in the JS sense, is always threatened by the capitalist or neo-liberal structures within which it is inescapably embedded. And, as we have seen, I cannot really engage with you as long as I am primarily operating to defend what I conceive myself to be and to bolster this through acquisition. In the play, the good-hearted prostitute Shen Te (Shanta in Ganguly's Bengali version) is forced to materialise her alter-ego 'protector'/cousin Shui Ta (>brother Shanta Prasad), but in so doing she undermines her own humanity, since 'he' is essentially a hard-nosed exploitative capitalist. This is difficult stuff for a Forum. But it is the kind of stuff Ganguly and JS do not shirk.

Some of the transpositions come naturally: Brecht's gods in quest of a 'good person' become Brahma, Vishnu and Shiva; and their debate about the likelihood of success is placed within contemporary Indian realities of life for the marginalised. The Water-Seller was, like one of the core team members, previously a hawker; the airman in Brecht's original becomes a taxi-driver. The play is set up as a challenge to 'the people' to respond to the situation the gods discover on their trip, that 'the lion's share is consumed by the few and the majority are suffering'. Moreover, they live in a context where:

SHIVA: Your entire creation has become adulterated today! Food, cloth-
    ing, shelter, everything!
BRAHMA: What is the administration doing about it?
SHIVA: Administration? That is a hub of corruption. Bribery, black mar-
    keting, all these are the norm there.
BRAHMA: How do you know all this?
SHIVA: Of course I know. It is these black marketeers who visit me every
    year chanting 'bhole baba paar karega' and pour water on me.
    (Ganguly, *Bhalo Manush*, tr. from Bengali by Sujoy Gangopadhyaya: sc. 1)

Goodness is difficult to come by in this scenario, and the people (read 'spectators') will need to 'make their own judgements about good and bad'. And they will need to be wary of many of those who claim to be on their side, not just the obviously powerful:

What about the so called 'activists' and 'social workers'. They are equally at fault, aren't they? It's in their interest to preserve these divisions. Unless society has problems, how will these people keep up their high standard of living? They are getting rich from other people's misery and blaming it all on religion and claiming to be progressive.

(Ibid)

So the play asks both moral questions about behaviour and self-reflexive ones about its own provenance. It also challenges actors and spectators with its length, and some experiments with shadow-play in the first performances were difficult to stage in the villages. The question this asks is 'can JS and their audiences navigate this kind of complex text and perceive its relevance to questions they face in their daily lives, in the same way as with short Forum plays?' Doing plays like this is a deliber- ate strategy to test the aesthetic, intellectual and critical capacity of the audiences JS has worked with over decades.

These 'new format' pieces did not replace the 'normal business' of doing Forum, training teams, creating plays and, as Chapter One has indicated, paralleling and interweaving this work with engagement in projects and continuing new ventures in community activity. Ganguly's recognition by the Ibsen Foundation through the award of a Fellowship in 2018 enabled JS to tackle another iconic 'western' play on an issue central to much of their work.

A DOLL'S HOUSE (KHELAR GHOR) (2018)

Ibsen's *A Doll's House* has been produced in Kolkata before, but this was the first time a Forum Theatre adaptation, in Bengali, had been attempted. The aim was to adapt Ibsen's *A Doll's House* to a Bengali context and address questions about patriarchy, especially in rural areas showing a high prevalence of patriarchal traditions.

This third adaptation from pre-existing plays is another bold combination of generic forms. Like *A Village Dream* and *The Good Person of Szechwan* before it, the adaptation of *A Doll's House* aims to do a number of things. Firstly, it positions one of the key issues which JS has addressed over three decades within an international context, but in so doing continues to affirm its direct relevance to Bengali realities. Secondly, it showcases Jana Sanskriti's complex and dynamic dramaturgy and signals – principally to audiences and the critical spectrum in India, since international reception has acclaimed it for a long time – the quality and innovation of JS's performance aesthetic. Thirdly, it enables JS to work with and welcome into its family young actors from the Kolkata area and introduce them to its methodology and goals. Funding attached to the Fellowship allowed JS to pay these new performers at rates in excess of those most 'established' Kolkata theatre companies offer.

Sanjoy Ganguly translated and adapted the text; his version uses an Ancient Greek-style chorus, part-speaking and partly producing still and moving images, to materialise much of the atmosphere and emotional subtext of the play; and draws on live music from the Bengali folk-form *jatra*. As always, in this production Ganguly's directorial method is co-creative: he involves the actors in creating text and images, working out what will go where and how they can contribute. The production developed through a series of workshops which wove together a mix of Indian forms, Boalian methods, psychopolitical scenarios, 'Greek' chorus-work and symbolic image-and-soundscapes.

The production aimed to create moments which speak, visually as well as verbally; to signal the complexity of the interactions and attitudes; not to close things down. The play ends with an open door; a question, not a solution, and thus provides a seamless shift into the Forum session. If Torvald Helmer (Hemanto or Hem in the Bengali version) is patently and pathetically patriarchal, even that posture is not without its complex causality; whilst for equally layered reasons Nora (now called Oporajita, Opa for short) is a problematic heroine who may, by the end, be beginning to recognise her own internalised oppression, but is a long way from 'solving' it.

A hundred years after the opening of Ibsen's play, Elfriede Jelinek wrote a play called *What happened to Nora after she left her husband?* (Jelinek 1984). Her Nora walks into a world whose gendered and economic parameters have not changed, and the play explores how she copes with them. The questions which both urban and rural Bengali audiences took on board, in performances which have occurred in a number of locations between 2018 and 2020, recognised these dimensions. Debate and interventions in Forum sessions has been particularly lively, and both JS's performance parameters and Ibsen's provocative

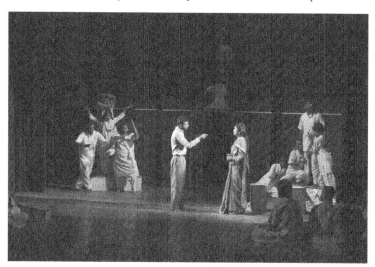

Figure 3.16 JS, *Khelar Ghor*: Bidyut (Krogstad in Ibsen) and Opa (Nora) with image-scape from chorus.

Photo: Jana Sanskriti

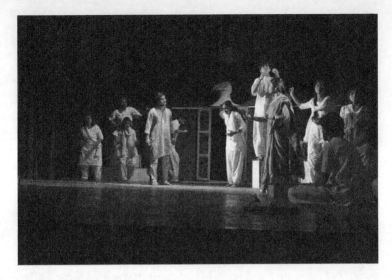

Figure 3.17 *Khelar Ghor*: Himobonto (Torvald), Shanti (maid), Opa (Nora) and
chorus.

Photo: Jana Sanskriti

text have played their part. In one of these sessions, Ganguly dealt with
the large number of people from the audience who wanted to intervene
by permitting a queue of spect-actors to line up on stage to replace the
protagonist and antagonist by turns! A Greek visitor who was present
also reported that, 'just to make it even more crazy, the chorus would
participate taking sides, sometimes on behalf of the protagonist, sometimes on … behalf of the antagonist, sometimes as an internal voice,
sometimes as the embodied voice of [a] social perspective'. The entire
audience, he says, was focused on the process (Kompogiorgas 2019).
JS's work continues to challenge and stimulate its public in many ways.

APPENDIX: LIST OF JANA SANSKRITI
PLAYS

1. JANA SANSKRITI'S MAJOR INTERACTIVE
AND FORUM PLAYS

1985 *Gayer Panchali* (Song of the Village)+*
1991 *Shonar Meye* (Golden Girl)*

1992 *Sarama*+
The Brick Factory (Ithbhata)+
1993 *Amra Jekhane Dariye* (*Where We* Stand)+*
2001 *Alas Liquor* (*Hayre Mod*) (on alcoholism)
2002 *Present Society* (*Bortaman Samaj*)
2002 *BPL* (*Below the Poverty Line*)
2004 *Terror* (*Sontras*) (on inter-party violence)
2007 *Drishtikon* (Perspective)+
2007 *New Agriculture* (*Natun Chash*) (on Monsanto and the effects of
        fertilisers)
2008 *Development* (*Unnayan*)
2009 *Education* 1 and 2*
2010 *Development 2* (on corporate intervention)
2012 *Trafficking* (*Bandona Theke Bindia*)
2013 *Investigation* (*Tondonta*) (on Subhash Chandra Bose)
2014 *The World of Minu* (on domestic violence)
2019 *The Story of Hadu* ('bad reputation')
2020 *Gaon Hatche Shohore* (*Villages Walking Towards Cities*)
        Porijayee Kene? (*Why Are We Migrants?*)

plus other short plays and scenarios
plus plays created in combination with associated groups, e.g. in Delhi,
Maharashtra, Orissa, Jharkand

- + = script in *Where We Stand* (2009, 2018)
- = 1000+ performances
- Between 1993 and 2001, JS was establishing and training local teams
  and developing work with them which subsequently fed into plays. It
  was also going through the process of establishing itself as an independent organisation and constructing its physical base (see Chapter One).
  In the period between 2014 and 2019 the core team was developing
  the plays mentioned below, as well as continuing to support regular
  performances of existing plays and variations in the rural areas.

2. EXISTING PLAYS TRANSLATED AND ADAPTED BY SANJOY GANGULY

2011 *The Village Dream* (Mesgun Zerai, Ethiopia)
2016, 2019 *The Good Person of Szechwan* (Bertolt Brecht)

2018> *A Doll's House* (Henrik Ibsen) (Ibsen Fellowship production: patriarchy in West Bengal)

All the plays listed under 1 above are originally in Bengali and many of them exist only in the form of handwritten notations or as drafts; those published in *Where We Stand* have been translated into English by Dia Da Costa. Those listed under 2 have been adapted and translated into Bengali by Ganguly, working from published translations from the original language into English. The Bengali adaptations of *Good Person* and *A Doll's House* have been translated into English by Sujoy Gangopadhyaya, but are only available as draft files.

4

WORKSHOPPING PRACTICES OF RELATIONSHIP

PARAMETERS AND GOALS

This chapter focuses on the exercises and activities which Jana San-skriti use in the development of performers. It looks at what kind of exercises they use, how they work with them and why they use them. From this it is possible to ask: how far are these examples and methods transferable to practitioners and situations in other places? Can the principles underlying them be 'translated' into other contexts and areas of work?

The exercises can be used to some extent as a toolkit. But in a workshop, between living, reactive, responsive human beings, the way things work affects what they are and what people derive from them. That means that sometimes the end-oriented goal needs to be suspended in order to 'listen' to what is actually occurring, or to allow confusion or difficulty to be given attention. The 'blocks' may some-times be vital parts of the work; engaging with them rather than pushing through them allows them to function as a springboard for new insights and kinds of response. Anyone who works with people in crisis and problematic situations needs to be alert to these dimensions, and JS's practice aims to assist with this.

DOI: 10.4324/9780429288753-4

Many exercises can be used for a variety of purposes, depending on the context. Here are some reflections on their use in TO by well-known practitioners:

'What do you use TO games for?'

   Cora Fairstein: 'If we want to be able to create, and to facilitate processes of creation in other people, when we want to imagine other possible realities and take them to a scene, playing games [is] a good start ... I use the games to generate trust, to bring attention to something in everyday life, to promote contact with one's own body in a new way ... that is, to de-mechanize.'

   'I always incorporate a game that allows me to visualize some relationship of power ...'

   Roberto Mazzini: 'to fight against oppressions at a bodily level [...] also as a preparation of needed skills for the Rainbow of Desire set of techniques ...'

   Birgit Fritz: 'because I believe in their revolutionary power ... to touch issues that might not be able to be verbalized ... to strengthen people's beliefs in their own abilities – and because [games] actually do create new realities and thus bring about change.'

   'The games serve as an alphabet for anything to come.'

(in Howe et al. 2019: 143–6)

At the beginning of workshops and in much of his work, Sanjoy Ganguly reminds people of the well-known spatial properties of a circle. Fritz notes that a workshop is a way to 'try to democratize the space' (ibid: 145), which may also involve the leader giving up some privileges – not least the claim to know or control what will happen, whilst recognising the responsibility to curate ways of negotiating what does. When people start to work with JS, they make a circle. They touch hands, or hold hands for a brief moment. They look at each other. There is no pressure. But just as Indian performers take off their shoes to enter the space (stage, house), there is a nod of recognition that 'we come together, here, now'. Usually then they are asked to walk. Ganguly calls it a 'circular walk', so its name still holds the idea of circle. Its form is looser: what it means is 'don't move in straight lines'. An opening quite familiar to many performers. But for anyone in the group who may feel uneasy, not too much of a threat. We are here; we can do this. Whatever this relationship is and wherever it will go, it starts by acknowledging everyone.

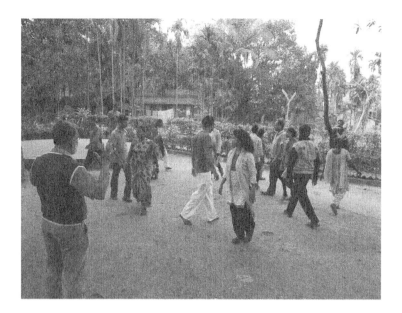

Figure 4.1 Jana Sanskriti core team initial walking exercise.

Photo: Jana Sanskriti

Ganguly's book *From Boal to Jana Sanskriti: Practice and Principles* (Ganguly 2017) presents six sets of exercises (about 30 exercises in total), illustrated by many photographs of the JS team doing them at Badu. In the book, only a small number of exercises are given under each section. In practice, Ganguly often spends between one and two hours on each exercise, exploring each one in depth, working intensively on each stage. This enables participants to explore many of the key transactions which take place in the creation of a Forum piece, and the kinds of interaction with other performers and potentially with spectators which may be required.

The work is directed towards:

- developing physical competencies and exploring ways of working interactively
- becoming familiar with the specific situations, conditions and processes of Forum
- acquiring particular skills to create character, dialogue and action in Forum scenarios

The first part of this chapter looks at selected examples in order to high-light the categories of work which JS uses and to investigate how they do it. In their case the focus is particularly on the *development of images towards the components of scenarios of exploitation, oppression and crisis* – as appropriate of course to the contexts of their work.

As with many approaches to acting, initial work concentrates on freeing up the resources of the body and the imagination, and getting people comfortable with working together.

The focus then shifts to the construction of images, which is interrupted and refocused by stages of reflection, analysis and identification.

From this a narrative for a scene or play begins to emerge which is fed back into and developed through further stages of work on move-ment, vocalisation and verbalisation.

The nuances and alternative configurations of characters, dialogue, point of view and action are then deepened and explored. The aim here is to create a rich and plausible representation of a lived reality which arises from a conflict situation and culminates in a crisis point.

Many of the exercises move through the following sequence:

individual body > shared image > collective image >
identification of situation > dynamisation > vocalisation >
reflection > elaboration

(The 'vocalisation' stage may be made up of several phases, e.g. the introduction of sound, key words, short sentences, inner mon-ologue and finally interactive dialogue, and may involve two or more participants, depending on the exercise.)

So they take participants along a path of experiencing, sharing, understanding and developing each step of a situation.

Many of the exercises also include *variations* which can be brought into play in order to open up the range of interactions and modalities which arise from the initial situation. The 'variation' template is a kind of open-ended pedagogy largely inherent in the 'games' approach to learning and to actor-training methodologies which use it; it is also specifically adopted by Boal as a signal of the (Freirean) 'dialogic' dynamic of his work, which JS enthusiastically embrace. Variation also implies further reflection on the how and why. In a workshop which Boal gave in India, a participant noted: 'He emphasizes analysing the game, understanding its process of working. This helps one to under-stand one's self, why one created a particular image, and in a broader perspective, also to understand others in respect to one's self' (Basak 1994: 30). This builds into the rhythm of the workshop *an alternation of action and reflection* which Ganguly identifies as fundamental to the whole Forum methodology.

The whole process of JS's work is both a form of improvised scene development and a training in working with (identifying, articulating physically and verbally, reflecting on and interrogating) the resources of each participant and the issues raised in the scene. This procedure is highly practical for performers who are invested in the material which forms the basis of the scenarios, since it is drawn from their own life experience; and who may not be familiar with or adept at reading or learning written scripts. Centrally, it engages the performers in creating their own world and offering it as a subject for debate.

The first essential goal of the exercises as JS uses them is to make Forum as good theatre.

This means discovering ways to train both fundamental acting skills and other capacities which are specifically related to acting in Forum. Underlying this are all the components which permeate JS's under-standing of both these dimensions, which have been outlined in the preceding three chapters.

In using the exercises it is important to remember that Forum:

- aims to pluralise, not to minimise, alternative visions, versions and kinds of investment
- is a 'game': different 'sides' get to play, using particular tactics, trying to achieve particular goals
- seeks to put in play the tactics and the stakes which underlie them so they can be evaluated
- is a space for dialogue and debate
- values problematising over solving
- seeks to enhance the confidence and competence of all players, onstage and offstage

The second essential goal is that the exercises should make sense as ways of lead-ing to the development of scenes which present aspects of the real-life situations of the performers and audience.

These two principles underpin all the work.

A JANA SANSKRITI TEMPLATE

From Boal to Jana Sanskriti sets out a sequence of exercises (itself of course a selection from a much larger range), starting with what at first seems to be a very simple 'walk', and leading through a variety of ways of interacting (both physically and verbally) in order to move towards the beginnings of scene construction. Many of the exercises JS use are found in their basic form in Boal's *Games for Actors and Non-Actors* (Boal 1992) and are themselves often imported from other methodologies and trainers. They all incorporate in some form the alternation of action and reflection which is central to all their work. Ian Watson notes that: '[t]he entire improvisation process is characterized as: **"observe-evaluate-react"**... [T]his process is also described as the development of a 'thinking act' (Watson 2001: 39; emphasis in original).

The following sections outline some of the sets and sequences of exercises which Sanjoy Ganguly regularly uses. The first part revisits many of the exercises shown in *From Boal to Jana Sanskriti*. They are described in bullet-points, illustrated by occasional photographs and diagrams, which aim to clarify the key processes and goals. A brief look at some examples from a workshop Augusto Boal gave in India himself opens up some similarities and comparisons with JS's workshop methodology. This helps to establish how it uses key TO techniques/processes/understandings in order to construct successive phases of introducing complexity in the development of script and performance, including aspects of Boal's Rainbow of Desire and Cop-in-the-Head processes to elaborate and develop characters and their interaction in scenes.

Exercises can be used in many ways. So, just as Boal adapts from other trainers and JS adapt from Boal, different aspects of an exercise can be employed for different purposes. But running through all of them are the following categories and goals:

- *warm-up*: e.g. 'walking'; 'Hello Harry'
  - Goals: fun, collaboration, interplay, loss of inhibition
- *interactive procedures:* e.g. mirroring, Colombian Hypnosis, pairs creating sculptures
  - Goals: observation, reaction and response, working together
- *stop/go, freeze-frame*
  - Goals: creating striking images, exploring rhythms, kinetics

- *improvisation*: role-play work, using 'Cop-in-the-Head' and 'Rainbow of Desire' processes
  - Goals: developing 'back-story', development and complexification of character, motivation, narrative
- *metaxis*: 'games as social metaphors': 'Glass Cobra'/Trade Union game; 'Granny's Footsteps'; 'The knot'
  - Goals: using fiction to understand reality, reflecting on the 'why' whilst doing
- *scripting*: storytelling (back-to-back or in small group); group devising
  - Goals: establishing context, scene, interaction and dramatic structure

The first set in *From Boal to Jana Sanskriti* is headed **Introductory Exercises**. These exercises all start to develop facility with body/feeling/expressivity/text and to practise ways of moving between them.

Unless otherwise indicated, participants should work without talking for the most part (except where they are specifically asked to share, discuss etc.).

Many of the exercises also build phases of recognition and reflection into the process; and it is often useful to have a short feedback in between exercises.

1. THE INITIAL WALKING EXERCISE

The *initial walking exercise* (Ganguly 2017: 3–5) is both familiar from quite a few other contexts and functions as a launching pad for much work; the 'circular walk' is used recurrently in JS's plays, as a way of either starting or of breaking a scene.

- Participants form a circle and acknowledge each other.
- The facilitator invites everyone to walk anywhere in the space, in any direction except straight lines and angles.
- On a clap from the facilitator, everyone freezes (each of the next steps is signalled by a clap).
- The facilitator invites each participant to choose a bird or animal and use their body to represent it, as precisely and expressively as possible.

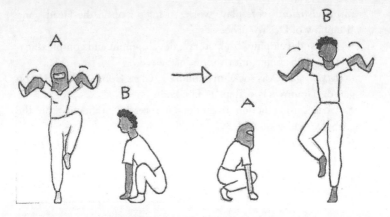

Figure 4.2 Swapping images.

Credit: Zorya Yarrow

- As the bird or animal, they move round the space; they can develop the animal as they move.
- On the next clap, they get into pairs, show each other their images and swap them (A>B, B>A).
- They do this with each other participant they meet, until all images have been exchanged.
- Then they look for the performer who is showing their original image.
- They pass to them the image they are currently embodying and leave the space.

Note: It's best if there are an even number of players and each one chooses a different animal or bird. The facilitator needs to be alert to suggest adjustments as necessary. If there is an odd number of players, one person won't be able to swap images at the end, so they keep the one they have.

The exercise serves as gentle warm-up, but it also begins to stimulate the imagination, to develop a sense of play, to encourage keen observation and to start the process of sharing and exchanging. The initial walking should aim for a relaxed alertness and an openness to whatever may occur.

2. FEEL THE PROTAGONIST

Feel the Protagonist (Ganguly 2017: 5–7) uses bodies to express feelings, develop observation and reaction.

- Participants form small groups (e.g. 4–6 people).
- Each person thinks of a situation of oppression.
- They share their examples with their groups.
- The groups each decide which can be best shown as a collective image.
- Each group constructs the chosen image with their bodies.
- *Variation*: the person whose image is chosen 'sculpts' the other participants into the image as s/he sees it.
  - *This sequence will need up to 15 minutes.*
- Groups then form pairs of groups with one group observing the other's image and creating another in response (each actor responds individually and then they are combined).
- Groups keep swapping until they have all observed and responded to each other.
  - *Responses should be quite rapid and spontaneous – within a maximum of 3 minutes.*

Note: *(i) The focus is on feeling and reacting, not analysing. The image should show how someone feels oppressed, marginalised, looked down on, unfairly treated etc. The response similarly physicalises an emotion.*

(ii): It is useful to keep in mind Julian (Augusto's son) Boal's definition of oppression as not just an individual relationship (though it may manifest itself as that), but 'a relation that benefits one group to the detriment of the other' (Fritz 2012: 103); there is also a social/political factor. The reflection afterwards can pick up on this.

3. EXPRESS EMOTION

Express Emotion (Ganguly 2017: 7–9) explores the range of expression, sets up a kind of 'Lightning Forum' situation, and moves between image and text. (In 'Lightning Forum', spect-actors offering different possible responses to a crisis-point line up and deliver a visual and/or verbal snapshot of their intervention one after another – at the end a general discussion evaluates which might be the best to pursue further.)

- Actors form two lines about 10m apart, facing away from each other but having identified a partner opposite.
- The facilitator gives each line a different emotion (anger, bewilderment, anxiety etc.).

- The actors in each line individually make an image of the emotion, using their faces and bodies.
- On the facilitator's clap, they turn and face the other line.
- One at a time, a pair walks towards each other and exchanges the emotion as they pass.
- The receiver incorporates as much as possible of the facial and bodily characteristics as they progress towards the other side of the space.

Variation: the two lines make an image of an oppressor and an oppressed character and repeat the exercise, but only to the point where the pair of characters is close to each other. Then they start to improvise a dialogue until the facilitator claps and they freeze in an image. Following this, the 'lightning' sequence has all other actors replace the protagonist in the dialogue phase for about a minute each, and then each one is discussed.

Note: *the images may be quite simple: one hand raised may evoke any number of bodily and facial reactions from the partner. Again the point is not to examine oppression intellectually at this stage, but to register and respond spontaneously.*

4. INDIAN PARLIAMENT

Indian Parliament (Ganguly 2017: 9–10) focuses on the use of language; it requires rapid improvisation of confrontational dialogue from representatives of different parties (the Indian National Assembly is renowned for 'out-of order' spontaneous verbal – and sometimes more than verbal – confrontations on the floor of the House). As well as reflecting a fairly ubiquitous political reality in an amusing way, this exercise sharpens awareness of verbal and visual cues and tones up intellectual reactions, drawing on traditions of repartee found in many Indian folk forms, which include debating in verse. However, it's not important to reproduce the specifically Indian characteristics, but to find parallel processes in your own context. So to use this game in another cultural context, try the following:

- Invite suggestions of a current political issue ('political' in a broad sense).
- Set up a 'formal' space for debate (e.g. participants construct a 'boxing ring' with their bodies).
- Invite volunteers to take on two (or more) positions in the debate/ argument.

- Determine a time allocation (e.g. two minutes for each speaker).
- Run an initial scenario as a verbal sparring match; onlookers may applaud/support vocally.
- Invite a second 'cast' to rerun the scenario, sharpening the interaction and employing any culturally appropriate relevant verbal/vocal strategies (e.g. rap, rhyme, song).
- The group divides into small groups of 2–4 and repeats the exercise, so that everyone gets the chance to play.

*Note: focus on **listening** to the argument and **responding** swiftly. It is less important to 'win' the argument than to play with ways of working with it, seeing possibilities of expanding the interaction.*

5. FISH SOCIETY

Fish Society (Ganguly 2017: 10–12, like many JS exercises, starts off as a simple and amusing physical encounter, but takes participants into further kinds of exploration.

- Participants walk around the space.
- The facilitator selects two actors and positions a ball between their mouths.
- These two players resume moving slowly, making sure they do not drop the ball.
- All the other players then come together like a shoal of fish and collectively try to reach the ball ('fish food') with their mouths; not surprisingly, this is very difficult.
- After playing this for some time (e.g. 3–5 minutes), participants are asked individually to find a single word which represents what they are feeling.
- Then they divide into small groups and share their words (they can write them on a flipchart or share verbally).
- Each group selects one of the words and forms a collective image of it.
- Each group shows their image to the others.

Note: on one level this is a group sensitivity/cohesion and de-inhibiting exercise; it then moves to identify emotional experience and find a way in which it can be represented collectively. Its trajectory is: **action > emotion > reflection > expression**.

6. GAME OF POWER

Game of Power (Ganguly 2017: 13–15) is rather different from Boal's 'Great Game of Power' (Boal 1992: 150), which asks actors to enter a space one by one and place themselves in the most powerful position, though it similarly addresses status.

- Form a circle.
- Number off from 1 to 7, so seven different levels are available.
- Each actor turns away from the others and creates an appropriate character depending on the value s/he has been allocated (1 = low, 7 = powerful).
- When they have found a character, participants raise a hand.
- When everyone is ready, the facilitator asks them to turn round and start to each portray their character, at first non-verbally: they don't interact with other participants, but can engage with one or more invisible/imaginary characters to show the situation more clearly.
- When prompted by the facilitator, each actor in character begins to speak to their imaginary invisible characters.
- When prompted, they start to speak to the other characters in the space.
- Everyone has to interact with all other participants for up to two minutes at a time.
- This means that all levels interact with each other.
- When this is complete, the facilitator puts participants in groups so that each group has characters from all strata in society.
- Each group then makes an image of power in society, using the characters they have established.

*Note: In this exercise, performers engage in successive phases of relationship with other participants via mime, monologue and verbal interaction. The work is firstly on finding and deploying physicality as expression, then increasingly on interaction and response, with a focus on negotiating different levels and positions of power. The sequence here is again **from emotion to image to text**. In addition, the exercise moves players towards recognising and negotiating different kinds of social reality in appearance and in speech. So it can and should last for quite a long time, and can also profitably lead into reflection and discussion about what people have experienced and noticed.*

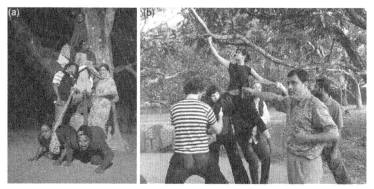

Figure 4.3 a) The Game of Power (JS core team members); b) The Game of Power (Muktadhara workshop).

Photos: Jana Sanskriti

If the group in total is smaller than seven, or the total number is not a multiple of seven, the facilitator may adjust the number of levels – though at least five is advisable. With a small number of participants the last but one step is omitted.

7. EXPRESSION WITH BODY

4.7. *Expression with Body* (Ganguly 2017: 15–16) uses a blank mask or piece of cloth to conceal the face and asks performers to express their situation with the body. Similarly to some of Lecoq's neutral mask work, removing the channel of facial expression is intended to dynamise the body.

- A performer puts on a mask and is given a character sketch and scenario by the facilitator (without other participants hearing).
- They are asked to portray all the emotions of the situation whilst wearing the mask (i.e. without recourse to most aspects of facial expression).
- Another performer is invited to enter as the ally or antagonist of the first.
- They play out a scene in mime which develops the story, without words.

Note: *These exercises aim to stimulate emotional, physical and verbal response. They are ways of starting the process by which performers will be increasingly able* *to offer visual, rhythmic and verbal cues to an audience about how a situation is affecting the characters involved. They need for the most part to be done quite slowly, not rushed. Try to explore rather than 'get it right' (there is no 'right').*

When Ganguly says that a sequence is not necessary (17), he means the exercises don't need to be done in a set sequence. People can develop their own compilation, or change some (cultural) elements. But it is useful to look out for what the work is aiming to do in each exercise and to recognise that different kinds of capacities are being put in play by them. The basic set begins to lay out the structural spine of the work as JS practises it. The main planks, which will recur later, are:

IMAGE > PLURALISATION > INTERACTION > DYNAMISATION >VOCALISATION

The last phase (vocalisation) often progresses through:

SOUND > KEY WORDS > SENTENCES > INNER MONOLOGUE > DIALOGUE

Something happens to your character. You utter a sound/sounds. You start to spit out nuggets of language, then progressively to string sentences together and finally to interact with someone else.

FIVE WORKSHOPS

The next section of the book details five workshops.

WORKSHOP 1

Workshop 1 (Ganguly 2017: 19–32) consists of three exercises and one additional variation. They share a common structure:

- an image, derived from movement or emotional response, is produced by individuals and pairs
- a group or combined image is formed from this
- the collective image is observed, described and named

The 'abstract' image is shifted towards a 'concrete' meaning from which the beginnings of a plot or narrative can emerge.

8. JOINT SCUPLTURE

In *Joint Sculpture*, everyone starts walking round the space, then the facilitator gives instructions as follows:

- walk > freeze > walk
- increase speed ('you are catching a train/plane')
- stop
- join hands with people nearest to you
- stretch bodies so that everyone is part of a group image
- half the group remains in the image, the other half leave and observe
- observers name image > say what it shows > tell its story

Note: be available/be in touch/stretch to your limit/support others/examine what you are producing. These are principles of relationship, co-production and scrutiny/problematisation which will serve much of the work to come.

9. CIRCLES OF EMOTION

Circles of Emotion begins from embodied exploration of basic emotions.

- Set this up by marking the names of six to eight emotions (love, anger, pride etc.) in zones on the floor/ground (e.g. in chalk) around the outside of the space.
- Participants walk in a circle, passing through each of the zones in turn.
- On the facilitator's clap they freeze, observe which zone they are in, and instantly adopt a body position and facial expression to express the relevant emotion.
- One person volunteers to group three or four of the images together to suggest a story.
- The remaining participants have to offer a title for the story and try to narrate what is happening.

*Note: Performance theorist Richard Schechner calls the initial phase of this 'rasa boxes': the ancient Indian performance manual **Natya Sastra** classifies nine fundamental emotional states called rasas – 'tastes' or 'flavours' – and details ways of training performers to demonstrate them. This 'freestyle' version encourages play with the relationship between felt emotion and physical expression.*

10. SCULPTING IN PAIRS

Sculpting in Pairs begins with a Boal exercise: players choose a partner and one person ('the artist') makes a sculpture with the body of the other ('the clay'), with as much precision and detail as possible – paying attention to the direction and angles of limbs, fingers etc., to the direction of the gaze and to facial expression. The 'sculptor' should not speak but signal or mirror what they are aiming for; they may move limbs gently, but can also work without touching if that is an issue. The 'sculpture' should be as pliable as possible during the process and then hold the position and expression for a short while when the 'work' is completed.

- Then they swap and repeat the exercise.
- Then everyone shows what they have been sculpted as, whilst also observing all the other sculptures.
- One person volunteers, or is asked to compose a group image, using several sculptures (say between 3 and 6); the rest of the group has to choose a story to describe it, which should be as close to real experience as possible.
- The people who were part of the group image become spectators whilst everyone else, including the group-image sculptor, takes up their original sculpted image again.
- The group image > story sequence is repeated.
- As far as numbers permit, groups swap around until everyone has been part of the group image and part of the group who has to describe it.

A *variation* gets one person from each pair to sculpt a detailed image of an oppressive situation they have witnessed:

- The 'artists' go to the side and observe the sculptures.
- Then they sculpt themselves as the oppressor in their image.
- On a clap, pairs start to act out the story: all in mime so far.
- They continue to improvise until the facilitator claps and everyone freezes.
- One pair is asked to show whilst the others observe.
- Then they are asked to add sound (not words): Ganguly uses 'ooh-la-la' for this, having heard it during a workshop he was giving in France!

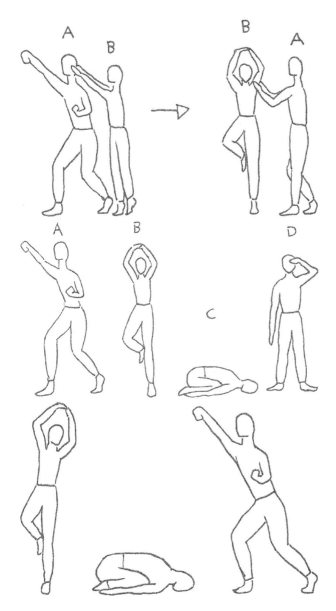

Figures 4.4, 4.5, 4.6 Sculpting in Pairs.

Credit: Zorya Yarrow

- On a clap, they freeze in an image.
- The audience narrates their story with help from the facilitator's prompts and questions ('what are their names/jobs?' 'what is the setting?' etc.).
- After several stories have been created, one is chosen: this one is further developed by improvising dialogue.
- Other images are subsequently also reworked in the same way.

Note: In this set of exercises:

- *exploration of body expressivity and feeling feeds into*
- *improvising scenes*
- which move out from *situation* to *emotion* to *physical expression* (body + face)
- and then to *action, vocalisation* and lastly *verbalisation*

The 'spine' here is:

CRISIS/CONFLICT > EMBODIMENT > ARTICULATION > INTERACTION

The latter stages begin to *explore alternative positions, both physical and verbal, in the conflict situation, and to introduce different possibilities as a spectrum of blocks and desires.* So the work has moved to the stage of *recognising, interrogating and problematising* the initial (image)-situation. This will be developed further by drawing on exercises based on Boal's Rainbow of Desire and Cop-in-the-Head work.

Note: Kelly Howe reminds facilitators of the need to be alert in exercises which involve physical activity and contact to the potential different abilities and sensitivities of people in the group. Parameters like race, gender and culture are not just concepts; they are embodied. 'To analyse power is the point of TO. That cannot be done in a vacuum-sealed environment. No space or practice is outside oppression' (Howe et al. 2019: 78). In JS's case, as noted in Chapter One, differences of caste and status often need this kind of attention.

The next sections of the book include exercises which become lengthier and more complex explorations, adding more levels of inter-action between people in groups. They develop the ability to register and respond emotionally and physically, sometimes individually, sometimes in connection with others. These exercises focus principally on feeling and expression as personal and interactive, but then also move into verbalisation.

WORKSHOP 2

Workshop 2 (Ganguly 2017: 33–52) has four well-known games and exercises, two of which are given here. The basic model is extended through a series of stages in which participants explore and reflect on increasingly complex implications of the images and situations they create.

11. 'HUMAN KNOT' EXERCISE

A variation on Boal's *'human knot' exercise* (Boal 1992: 67–8).
   The *basic form* is:

- participants join hands in a circle
- the facilitator may – or may not – ask them to close their eyes
- the facilitator guides them to interweave with each other, by stepping over or crawling under the joined arms
- without losing the grip, they try to untie themselves and recover the initial formation

In the *variation*:

- the facilitator asks the group to walk round very close to each other, using circular movements and weaving around and in between each other
- on a clap, they freeze
- each person joins hands with two others: right hand to left hand, left to right (no talking)
- everyone closes their eyes
- they are asked to imagine that they are trapped in this position
- with eyes closed, the group tries to untangle itself (the facilitator needs to ensure they don't risk hurting themselves)
- on a clap, they freeze
- they are invited to reflect on how they are feeling
- they open their eyes and continue to try to untie the knot
- if they don't succeed after a few minutes, the facilitator asks them to return to the original circle

- everyone closes their eyes
- everyone turns and faces outwards
- each person recalls the feelings they had during the activity
- each person makes an image to express these feelings
- when they are ready, they turn back into the circle, showing their images
- everyone opens their eyes and observes everyone else's image
- they make groups with people who have similar images
- the facilitator numbers the groups
- one group at a time shows its collection of images, whilst the others observe
- on a clap, they add movement (feet remain still)
- on another clap, each person in the group speaks a word or phrase which describes their feeling and keeps on doing so and moving for a short while
- then they write their words on a flipchart
- when all groups have done this, the facilitator creates new groups
- each group chooses a word or phrase from the flipchart
- they create a composite image using this stimulus
- the image should show an example of oppression
- it should have a story behind it, and the characters and situation should be clear
- groups show their image to the others
- the audience is asked to interpret each one
- groups then develop their image into a sequence of three still images which show how the story develops
- each group presents its sequence
- as it unfolds, an audience member chosen by the facilitator (or a volunteer) narrates the story in detail (like a football commentary) with names and relationships and as much precise information as possible

Note (i) *What is especially developed in the later phases of the 'knot' variation, is* **reflection, analysis and commentary**, *leading on to* **discovering multiple narratives which express different potential attitudes, emotions and perspectives**.

(ii) *This is an excellent example of Ganguly's practice of working with exercises. A relatively simple or well-known template is explored and extended in several ways, identifying and using experience to begin to create story and scenario. The exercise could easily last for several hours.*

12. GRANDMOTHER'S FOOTSTEPS

Two variations of the familiar game *Grandmother's Footsteps* (Boal 1992: 81).

The basic version:

* 'Granny' faces the front
* all other players start at a distance
* on the facilitator's clap, players start to move towards her in an attempt to touch her before she 'catches' them
* Granny may turn round at any moment
* when she does so, players freeze
* if Granny sees a player moving any part of the body, she calls them out and they have to go back to the beginning

(Players may be required to move independently or to form groups of two or three who must remain in tactile contact as they move together.)

The first variation (*Deer and Tiger*) describes the 'Granny' figure as a 'fascist tiger' and the other players as deer:

* the deer can 'kill' the tiger by touching it
* they should be ready to sacrifice their lives for the sake of 'democracy' in the wood
* the exercise is played as above

The second variation is called *Crossing the Border*:

* 'Granny' becomes a border guard
* players are divided into 'family groups' of three
* they try to escape (i.e. touching the border) without being caught (i.e. be seen moving)
* if the facilitator sees a striking image in any of the freeze moments, s/he can stop the game and invite the group to observe it
* the group is then invited to analyse and explore the meaning which they read into that image
* the meaning should be 'grounded in reality' (43)

Note: *The complications introduced here shift the game towards analysis of political situations. One develops working together as physical experience, the* *other encourages a political reading of an image, rather than just an interpersonal dynamic. JS thus tries to introduce 'politics' as a process and a recognition into what is usually played as a fun warm-up exercise.*

When you are in close contact, as in all of these games, tactile experience generates feelings – of connection or resistance, of comfort or discomfort, for example. If you add to that a collective task with a particular quality, another level of response is activated. In the 'Granny' exercise, it's initially about co-operation, both as a rapid and possibly silent exchange of impulses, and as a shared drive towards achieving a goal (reaching 'Granny' without being caught). The 'human knot' may generate more ambivalent emotions, since unravelling from the complicated knot may be difficult and frustrating – especially with eyes closed – and different people may move at different speeds. People may feel conflicting impulses, like 'I want to help', 'I am frustrated', 'I want to get out', 'if everyone follows me we can do it', and so on. So the ensuing reflection is a chance to note, interrogate and explore how this contact plays out physically and emotionally, and how different people feel in relation to themselves and to the group. In both these games, reflection and analysis is added to the mix, so that participants are working with bodies, emotions and intellect together.

WORKSHOP 3

Workshop 3 (Ganguly 2017: 53–67) has four exercises, of which three are described here. The exercises aim to continue the direction towards fleshing out more *variations of building up interaction and interrelationship* in scenarios. They work by multiplying the number of different versions and perspectives which can be located in any encounter and interrogated in a Forum session. Power dynamics can shift; a problem can be seen from several angles, which may imply different approaches to addressing it. This kind of work is a version of 'Stanislavskian' approaches to 'sub-text', in that it starts the process of *unpicking the different drives and attitudes* which impel the participants in any situation. In exercises where participants swap body images, roles etc., they are undergoing a training in experiencing how to see the world from another person's vantage point. They begin to embody this key skill, which is essential to the business of Forum.

13. FORUM IN A CIRCLE

Forum in a Circle specifically designates itself as preparation for the kinds of response, reaction and invention required when doing Forum, and aims to enable the actors to 'explore each problem in a different way each time' (Ganguly 2017: 56). This, as we have seen, is a crucial factor in the way JS work.

- Groups of three develop a short role-play (with text) based on a real oppression: one oppressor, one oppressed character, one person who tries unsuccessfully to help the latter.
- Working separately and simultaneously, each group perform the scene three times, swapping roles so that each performer plays each role.
- Each time they should attempt to find new dimensions in the conflict.
- Then develop it further (5–10 minutes to do this).
- They perform it to everyone.
- Then the protagonist in each scene moves to another group and the scene is played again.
- Once again, the 'new' group should look for new angles (e.g. the protagonist uses different tactics to try to change the situation).
- This move is then also repeated as many times as necessary.

14. COLOMBIAN HYPNOSIS

The next exercise is a variation on Boal's *Colombian Hypnosis* (Boal 1992: 63), where one player leads the other around with the palm of the hand close to their face. Ganguly emphasises the need to do this slowly, and pauses it at regular intervals so the pairs form an image.

- Then the facilitator chooses two or three images and asks other players to reflect on them, identify the power dynamics, suggest a situation and so on.
- After this everyone repeats step one: the sequence is action > reflection > action.
- Hypnotisers and hypnotised then form two lines, face away from each other, reflect on their experience, create an image to express it, and turn and show the images.

- Then they come into the centre in their original pairs, present the images and move from there into a dialogue which begins to sketch out a scenario.
- Another *variation* puts the group into threes, with one hypnotiser leading the other two, and gets them to swap at intervals so they all do each role.
- Then everyone returns to the circle and is asked to find one word to express how they felt. Everyone walks around and shares the word with others as they meet.
- Then, in groups of five, they select one word and create a group image to depict that situation; each group shows its image, others try to guess the word.

This very extended sequence of alternations of image-reflection-verbalisation asks players to *embody and explore feelings and investigate what they might signify*. It is pursued in exercise 15, Storytelling.

15. STORYTELLING

Storytelling (Ganguly 2017: 64–7) frequently figures, in one form or another, in Ganguly's Muktadhara workshop on 'Scripting the Play'. He thus designates it as a useful launching-pad for the collective construction of performance-texts.

- Groups of three sit back-to-back and one person narrates a real-life story related to exploitation or oppression.
- The listeners, who close their eyes, ask for clarification where necessary; then they swap roles.
- At the end they choose one of the stories.
- This is presented to the rest of the participants by a narrator, who keeps his/her hands behind the back whilst a second person, standing behind with arms extended forward through the narrator's armpits, produces appropriate arm and hand gestures; the third member of the group uses their body and face to mime any actions and characters in the story.
- The spectators are then asked to create images of what they've heard and seen, using each other as sculptures where appropriate; the original group of three is asked to judge which is most evocative of their story. (All groups do this in turn.)

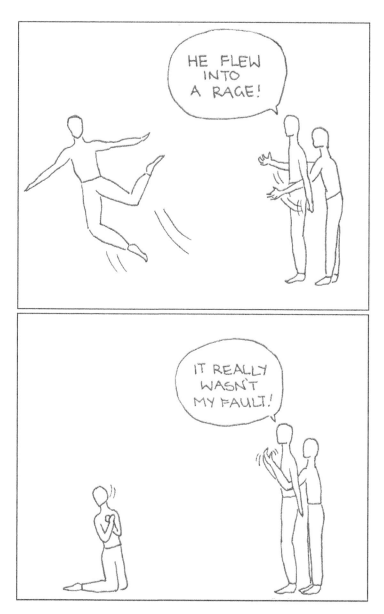

Figures 4.7, 4.8, 4.9 Storytelling in Threes.

Credit: Zorya Yarrow

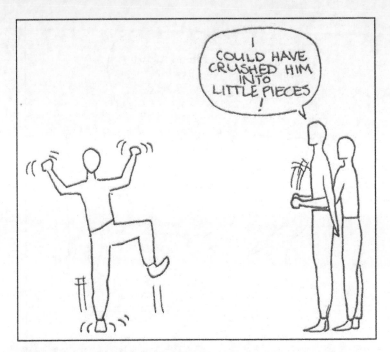

Figures 4.7, 4.8, 4.9 Continued

*Note: The exercise, constructed from different games which Ganguly encoun-
tered, emphasises the link between* **narration** *and* **embodiment**. *Like the others in this workshop, it practises the skills of* **identifying** *and* **articulating**
(physically and verbally) a **problematic or confrontational situation**,
and begins to explore how to **engage with and represent different ways
of understanding its causes** *and possible developments.*

Another way of looking at what occurs in using these exercises is to
note that they work with three dimensions of learning or pedagogical
process. The first of these dimensions is initially body-centred (motoric)
but also engages and stimulates cognitive activity; it includes:

* simple corporeal movement as the basis (motoric flexibility)
* group process development (eye contact, response and interaction,
  touching, creating shapes together)
* 'freeze-frame' practice (stop/go; action/image; event/significance;
  do/'read')

This combination of procedures:

- institutes dual-movement model (shifting between different rhythms and kinds of movement/activity)
- develops body/brain alternation
- instils a 'habit' of deconstructing/reconstructing

The next dimension brings together the cognitive and the affective (emotions and feelings):

- spontaneous response
- experiencing feelings
- recognising feelings
- recognising the dyad of feeling and action
- evaluating process spectrum

These action events are all quite 'basic'. But they cannot just be consigned to the category of 'low-level' performance training, although trained performers clearly have repertoires of more complex patterns. What they do is to engender *habits* of behaviour which become part of a repertoire, which includes recognising and analysing underlying social and behavioural patterns and structures; producing physical actions, and creating more complex scenarios in 'scripting the play'. They also lead onto further levels of the training process.

WORKSHOP 4

The group of exercises in **Workshop 4** (68–79) aims to develop *textures and levels of interaction* in the process of creating a scene. Examples include complex movement (Ex. 16) and attention to atmospheres (Ex. 19).

16. CATCH IN A CIRCLE

Catch in a Circle is concerned with movement and co-ordination.

- Participants make a circle and turn left.
- One person pushes the person in front and moves into the space left by them; the person pushed then does the same, so gradually the whole group begins to move in this way.

- Another person pushes someone two places ahead of them, and when they move, takes that place; that person then does the same.
- Now there are two different movements (and different rhythms) occurring at the same time – which could be coherent, chaotic or anything in between ...

17. HI HARRY – HULLO HARRY – BYE HARRY

A simpler but similar game (not in the book) is one JS also like to use. It's especially useful if working with groups who might initially be wary of or have different needs around physical contact.

Hi Harry – Hullo Harry – Bye Harry is a fast-paced 'starter' which also does a number of different jobs:

- everyone stands in a circle
- they number off sequentially up to 3 (1,2,3) and are allocated phrases
- Number 1s say 'Hi Harry'; No. 2s say 'Bye Harry'; No. 3s say 'Hullo Harry'
- but the phrases have to be spoken in the order given in the title: so as they progress round the circle the order of speaking is 1,3,2; 1,3,2
- thus No. 1 as it were 'touches' the person two spaces to the right vocally, who then 'touches' the person one space to the left, who then 'touches' the person two spaces to the right – and so on

Note: As the game progresses – say after one or two rounds – it should speed up. When the facilitator decides it is right, s/he announces that delay or failure means that person drops out. The game is usually hilarious and an excellent way to break ice and get across the message that 'failing' or 'getting it wrong' not only doesn't matter, but is actually beneficial for the game. This apparently fairly banal observation is in fact a key to psychological and pedagogical insights about the different processes of learning and being which can operate in this kind of work. This and other similar games are also valuable in negotiating status, hierarchy and internalised expectations about behaviour within groups, which is an important factor in JS's context too.

18. NEWSPAPER THEATRE

- Groups of four or five choose a story or picture from a paper and create a still image to represent the situation.

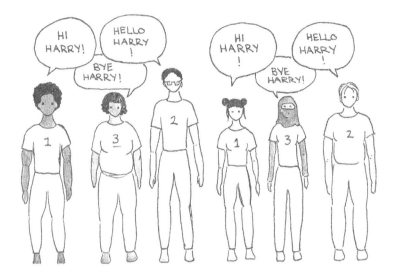

Figure 4.10 Hi Harry.

Credit: Zorya Yarrow

- They show their image to other groups.
- Each group pairs up with one other group.
- They observe each other's image and try to identify what the story is.
- They each create a new image to reflect their interpretation of what they saw.
- They extend this into a short mimed scene.
- All show their scenes, this time in stages: a) image; b) add movement; c) add text and sounds; d) everyone discusses what they have seen, heard and done.

Note: *This exercise incorporates the dimension of **deconstructing and reinterpreting** 'public reporting', and **developing a critical perspective** on mediatised information, whilst working with bodies and movement to materialise perspectives which may have been 'edited out' of the published text.*

19. SOUNDSCAPES AND IMAGES

- Groups of six are given 10 minutes to devise a soundscape (a storm, a train station, etc.).
- They perform it in sequence to all participants, who close their eyes.

- After each one, the listeners make a still image in their groups to reflect what they have heard.
- Each group shows its image.
- The whole group discusses what they interpreted from the soundscape.
- They work in groups to develop the soundscape further and repeat.

20. CHARACTERS' STORIES

- In the centre of the circle, place pieces of paper with the name of a role or function written on them (e.g. policeman, mother).
- Actors choose one and in groups of six compose a short silent scene which they then show; others guess who the characters are.

The examples which emerged from workshops with Jana Sanskriti performers are indicative of the spectrum of their work, e.g.: 'woman abandoned by husband'; 'bride on the way to wedding'; 'no one notices a rape'; 'a minister and the boss of an agribusiness cook up a deal'.

Note: Individual elements, contextual references, degrees of complexity etc. could be varied to suit different geographical, cultural and political circumstances. In House of Games, Chris Johnston presents a similar game ('The Sellotape Games') where participants move around the room with a post-it note on their back designating their character – which is initially unknown to them but they are asked to guess from other people's behaviour to them (Johnston 2005: 153).

WORKSHOP 5

The first two exercises in *Workshop 5* work again with images.

21. MOVING AS A STILL IMAGE

- Participants form a circle.
- They close their eyes.
- Everyone creates a whole-body image of oppression.
- Facilitator claps: they start to move around carefully, keeping their eyes closed and only moving their feet.
- Clap: they feel for other participants and form groups of five or six.
- Clap: they open their eyes and show others in the group their images.

- Each group chooses one of the images.
- Each group creates a silent scene arising from it, taking about 15 minutes to do this.
- These stories are then shown, shared and critiqued, examining the presentation and what it shows in detail.

Note: The first part of the exercise 'increases special awareness and concentration' (80): it uses tactile and psycho-physical processes and aims for detailed exploration, which feeds into the rest of the exercise.

22. EXPERIENCING THE LIVES OF OTHERS

- In a circle, facing outwards, participants imagine someone they know.
- When they are ready, they turn round and create an image of this person.
- The facilitator claps: they move round the space.
- When they meet another participant, they swap images.
- The exercise progresses by each participant taking on every image in turn and exploring it for several minutes at a time.

*Note: These exercises offer the chance to explore at some length the ways in which body image and expression can be closely experienced and studied as signifying practices. Like most of the other games and exercises outlined here, what may appear simple and unilinear may change its effect when done slowly, repeatedly and with frequent intervals of reflection. These two exercises take even further the attention to **image** and **emotion**, which has been important in others. Spending a long time working through stages of encountering, recognising, critiquing and representing emotional experience helps to familiarise participants with complex processes and gain the ability to negotiate them; very close attention to the development and production of images, individually and in groups, develops the ability to maximise the presentation of situations and to make possible the kinds of arresting visual representations which characterise JS's plays.*

Most of the exercises build this possibility of slowness into their process. Birgit Fritz says that she had the impression that Boal used to work like that at one time, and that 'with Sanjoy Ganguly's way of doing the games we start to rediscover what benefits time can actually bring us.' And in an acute observation which relates to both the political and the psychological dimension of these exercises, she notes that '[d]oing games with too little time can be an escape route, avoiding confrontation with awkward issues' (in Howe et al. 2019: 149).

It is in this light that it is useful to look at the final game in the book. As Eugene van Erven identifies, JS's adaptation of Boal's *Glass Cobra* turns it into a more complex socio-political experience. (For other descriptions, see Boal 1992: 108, and Frost & Yarrow 2015: 164). Van Erven notes that 'the game turned into an extended analytic exploration of relations in the workplace', marked by '[a] refusal to be rushed, [a] gentle insistence to dig ever deeper and consistently investigate new angles' (van Erven in Ganguly 2017: xi).

23. THE TRADE UNION GAME

- In a circle, participants turn right and feel the head, neck and shoulders of the person in front.
- The facilitator explains that they are members of a union.
- They are asked to close their eyes.
- Then the facilitator moves them one by one to different positions in the space, informing them that they have become divided, and support different parties or positions.
- The task then is to reconnect: each person needs to find the one who was in front of them and thus reform the circle, still with eyes closed. (This can take a long time!)
- When (or if) they come back together, they are all asked to open their eyes and discuss what they felt, whilst relating it to 'society'.

Note: The last phase of individual and collective consideration is given particular importance. This game, in Ganguly's reworking, functions as an experiential demonstration and thus a reflective recognition of what it feels like to be 'workers bewitched by commodity fetishism, divided by the competition, atrophied physically and mentally ...' (Soeiros & Boal in Howe et al. 2019: 96). It also of course materialises what occurs when each person pursues their own goals (though they may not have been fully consciously chosen).

This is also a kind of parallel to the 'human knot' game. Both set up situations of (tactile) relatedness, intensified by closing the eyes, and explore how this – physical and motoric –experience, modified in different ways (knotting up or breaking apart) directly feeds into affective or emotional behaviours. When performers are asked to think sociologically about this, a further level of transaction and interrelation is

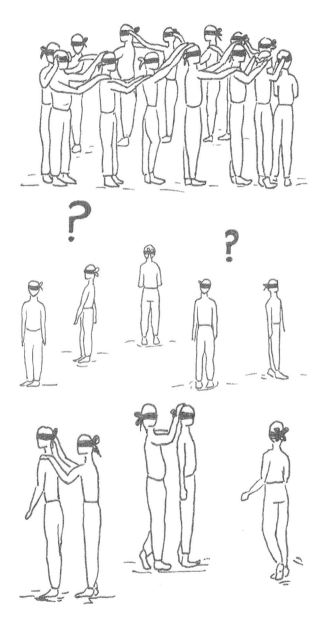

Figures 4.11, 4.12, 4.13 The Trade Union game.

Credit: Zorya Yarrow

activated, and helps them in the job of understanding how these factors interact in any personal or communal situation. Who I am, what I feel, how I understand, how I behave, what I think and say, and how I evaluate and communicate all of this with others, is the bodily and emotive subtext of the political, and both affects and is affected by it.

Throughout this section I have tried to indicate some of the methodology and goals of the exercises, as well as giving a brief description of them. At the same time, even including this and using diagrams to offer another way of understanding how they work, it's difficult to give a sense of the element of 'time'; that is perhaps particularly the case because I have also been concerned to show that JS always relates its training process to specific and material outcomes. Just as Ganguly recognised the need to 'think' in a different way in order to begin to connect with the people he wanted to work with, so his practice of doing exercises involves a kind of deconstruction of the 'end-oriented' mode which often creeps into workshops. Sometimes that is because the facilitator or leader is, under the various pressures of professionalisation and instrumentalism, driving towards a particular 'product' or set of results. But even where this isn't the case, it's often difficult for a facilitator (like a Joker) to be prepared to really engage with what is happening in the space between the people there and to put on hold his or her 'menu' of desired outcomes and stages by which to move towards them. Nor is it the case that JS facilitators, including Ganguly, always manage this. But this openness is at least as important as knowing what the exercises are and what order to do them in. That's why Ganguly says 'sequence isn't important' and why he, and Boal, and lots of other good actor-trainers, know that flexibility and attention to particular circumstance is a vital ingredient.

OTHER WORKSHOPS, INTERACTIVE DIMENSIONS AND TECHNIQUES

Boal himself conducted a workshop organised by Jana Sanskriti in India in 1994, which is documented in *Seagull Theatre Quarterly* (Basak 1994). In addition to JS, some ten other groups from across India participated. Twenty-five games are described, plus an account of a series of exercises from Boal's Rainbow of Desire methodology, interspersed with interviews with Boal, a Q and A session, and reflections from the author, Jhuma Basak.

Exercises with a similar structure to the JS models described above include the 'pilot/co-pilot', where one partner tells the story of a real event and the other listens, after which both create images to express their experience; a two-person oppressor-oppressed scenario which is built up gradually as facial expression > body image > use of space > addition of sound > words; and a short sketch of a typical 'couple' scenario. The group also encountered the game Boal calls 'The Revelations of St Theresa' (Boal 1992: 159–60) in which partners are allotted roles (e.g. husband/wife) and start an improvised scene into which each has to drop an unexpected and disturbing secret about the other. This also starts to move actors towards the territory of what Stanislavsky would call the 'sub-text', where material which is initially suppressed begins to be revealed and produces an effect on the relationship which is being sketched out.

The dramaturgical aim here is to get performers to craft increasingly complex interactions. Although Boal's 'psychological' strand of work (Rainbow and Cop-in-the Head) is often characterised as having arisen from a recognition of forms of oppression ('western' or 'internal') different from the overt presence of military agents of a despotic government in which Boal's work was developed, it has been widely used as a way to develop scenes by helping actors to envisage different facets of their characters.

Here are two exercises which JS has extrapolated from Boal's method and use frequently in workshops and scene development. They often figure in Ganguly's 'Scripting the Play' sequence.

24. CREATING SUB-TEXT: IMAGE>MONOLOGUE>DIALOGUE

- Run the essentials of a scene familiar to the participants.
- The actors who are not playing the two main characters make images to express different aspects of protagonist and antagonist (up to six for each): what are they feeling/thinking? (no words).
- The actors who played the protagonist and antagonist stand and observe.
- Arrange actors in pairs opposite each other, keeping their images intact – one line for protagonist, one for antagonist.
- Ask each actor-image to produce and deliver their own internal monologue (this could be developed in stages: utter a sound; speak a key word or words; extend these into a monologue).

- Each pair (one pair at a time) then engages in dialogue, building on the monologues they have spoken/heard.
- The original protagonist and antagonist take up the scene again and feed any of the images and dialogue they have observed into the developing script as appropriate (in other words, the actors playing the protagonist and antagonist have to note all the variations and use any or all of them as appropriate in successive runs of the scene).

Variation/extension:
- create internal monologue > dialogue for each character which expresses:
- their intentions/desires
- the blocks/resistances 'cops-in-the head' which prevent them realising these

25. PLURALISING CHARACTER

- Actors play an already created scene.
- Then the actors create different versions of each character.
- All actors swap roles and play scene again.
- Keep doing this until each actor has played all roles.
- Original actor for each character then needs to remember the different possibilities and use them to build up a more complex version.

SUMMARY AND FURTHER DIMENSIONS

Jana Sanskriti has been able to pick up all the potential implications of this work as a way to assist practice when working on the relationship between actor and character. These start from relatively familiar actorly skills of engaging with emotional dynamics, but also extend to aspects which are particularly relevant for actors in Forum and especially for the 'intervention' section: they include finding how to achieve a balance of emotion/reason, engagement/detachment and action/reflection.

TO training needs to cement the links between emotion memory, affective sub-text, embodied expressivity and the interaction of personal and social/political realities. Here it is useful to remember a further dimension of JS's orientation. Ganguly says:

> So basically, Boal's method is about opening doors; enlarging, magnifying the reality so they can discover the tiny elements within it. In the training which helps the performers to be able to identify and script their reality, we also use games and exercises as social metaphors; they are a bridge between participants inside the room and the reality outside. So people explore and cultivate their reality, they discover what is oppression, who is the oppressor, how do the oppressed think; they are either submissive or they want to protest. So our theatre workshops become a sociology class. Actors understand, before they go to the audience, they analyse the problem from a social science point of view. So that is why even the process is very important in TO. People often neglect the process, but it is, if not more than, equally important as the product.
>
> (Ganguly 2017: 91)

So in JS's practice, both as training and as performance, there is always a close correlation between these levels, and Rainbow of Desire and Cop-in-the-Head work is used:

- to emphasise that the individual is not separate from society
- to clarify that introspection is 'a mode of social observation'
- to assist women's groups (and many others) to identify inculturated patriarchy (Ganguly 2010: 124–5)
- to interrogate multiple dimensions and possibilities of oppressors and oppressed
- to animate or dynamise interactions and characters, both protagonist and antagonist and the 'bystander' characters
- to 'difficultate', complexify and stratify the developing performance-script

All of these features are part of a training for performers, Jokers and, ultimately, spect-actors in the Forum process. They help to ensure that Forum productions do not subside into wish-fulfilment or blaming, but function as careful and rigorous animations and investigations.

In 1997–8, as part of a project organised by Seagull called Theatre for Change, Jana Sanskriti led a workshop with Swayam, a crisis centre for abused women in Kolkata. *STQ* 20/21 (1998/9) includes a report on the workshop, accounts of subsequent discussion sessions with participants, facilitators and organisers, and the script of the play which emerged from the work and was performed on International Women's Day in 1998 in Triangular Park, Kolkata. The play itself is a kind of parallel to JS's *Shonar Meye* (see Chapter Three), into which material drawn from the lives of the women who created *Eije, Ami Ekhane* (*Look, Here I Am*) was incorporated.

Reliving some of these situations will not have been comfortable. The women who participated were enabled to do this and to turn that experience into a play which they presented with great pride. But nothing was ever taken for granted in the transaction, either during the workshopping process or on the occasion of the delivery. It is a territory of risk.

Recognising risk can open the door to a preparedness to remain with the difficulty. Sanjoy Ganguly is clear that in addition to being an effective method for actors of finding more resonances in a scene, using Rainbow techniques in Forum means encountering and negotiating things that it is easier to run away from. Chapter Two describes some work with a boy called Bakam, who lives in poverty with an often drunk father, who has other children by two sisters. Bakam's own process is explored in a Rainbow session in which he comes face to face with his desires (to strike out; to run away ...) and with the battle with the socialised will which would censor them. The other members of the group recognise the situation; some of them are able to dynamise the images of desire which Bakam had concurred with. But in so doing, Ganguly says, the individuals and the group went through their own journey: from empathy (understanding but not identifying with), to sympathy (feeling the situation as their own), to a kind of co-substantiality (being engaged together in the process of materialising it) (Ganguly 2010: 47–52). That is to say, the conjunction of Rainbow of Desire and Forum has to engage with the interface of the social, the personal/emotional and the mechanics of collective support in practice. This can be difficult and painful, embarrassing and uncomfortable. It needs time, but also the engagement of the whole group in the way Ganguly has described it. At a subsequent evaluation meeting between *STQ* and *JS*, Sanjoy Ganguly said: 'in the kind of work we do, group building is very important [...] We knew that they were not going to trust us so quickly and easily. They do not trust each other, why should they trust us?' If you undertake this work you need to be prepared on one hand to tune into the group in this way, and on the other hand not to run away, for example into over-hasty acquiescence with a proposal implied in an intervention which it is easy to agree with.

Forum can become formulaic. Dramaturgically and aesthetically it's the greatest danger, and one which has been extensively discussed among TO practitioners. One of the key reasons for this is the difficulty of engaging with difficulty! In a way that's no different from the need to work in detail on almost anything, and certainly on developing an argument or creating a piece of art. So here too, JS offers not only a 'what' but also a 'how' in the kinds of process it uses in facilitating workshops and delivering training.

FROM HERE TO WHERE?

In particular, Jana Sanskriti's work demonstrates that TO is not just a bunch of exercises or techniques. The focus of their practice of performance is to bring together theatre techniques, imaginative dramaturgy and collective creativity – both Indian and global – to forge new habits, structures and action. In so doing they fashion and nurture an art of relationship which is challengingly and pragmatically societal and political, and responsively and responsibly interpersonal, and which constitutes a dialogue of human resource in action. Encountering their work is a challenge, not to imitate but to think through the reasons for and processes of doing theatre, doing TO and being human. In and through it, 'the body becomes a space for hope' (Da Costa 2010: 626).

JS's practice is, across many dimensions, a way of raising questions as well as offering some answers. The answers from its work will not all be applicable in other geographical, political and historical circumstances. But JS's history and development, aims, goals and methods, and the results of that activity in terms of plays, training processes, engagement with communities and international presence, may provide some useful responses. They are not prescriptive. JS itself has changed as it has developed. It faces new challenges all the time, not least in an India in which communalism, factionalism, the politics of division and the evidence of gross economic disparity are all writ large. JS makes theatre as a response to that scenario. In so doing it has met with Boal and taken his work on, exemplifying and fulfilling many of its fundamental goals. So the exercises, like the processes of training and performance in which they are embedded, are an invitation to explore a politics of the fully human.

BIBLIOGRAPHY

Babbage, Frances (2004) *Augusto Boal*. London: Routledge.

Bala, Sruti and Albacan, Aristita I. (2013) 'Workshopping the Revolution? On the phenomenon of joker training in the Theatre of the Oppressed', *Research in Drama Education: the Journal of Applied Theatre and Performance*, 18(4), pp. 388–402.

Basak, Jhuma (1994) 'The theatre games of Augusto Boal: a workshop diary', *Seagull Theatre Quarterly*, 2, pp. 22–41.

Biswas, Bulbuli and Banerjee, Paramita (1997) 'Street theatre in Bengal: a glimpse', *Seagull Theatre Quarterly*, 16, pp. 31–7.

Boal, Augusto (1979) *Theatre of the Oppressed*. London: Pluto

Boal, Augusto (1992) *Games for actors and non-actors*. Translated by Adrian Jackson. London: Routledge.

Boal, Augusto (1995) *The rainbow of desire*. Translated by Adrian Jackson. London: Routledge.

Boal, Julian and Soeiro, José (2019) 'Identities, otherness, and emancipation in the Theatre of the Oppressed', in Howe, Kelly, Boal, Julian and Soeiro, José (eds) *The Routledge companion to Theatre of the Oppressed*. London & New York: Routledge, pp. 94–103.

Bogad, L.M. (2006) 'Tactical carnival: social movements, demonstrations, and dialogical performance', in Cohen-Cruz, Jan and Schutzman, Mady (eds), *A Boal companion: dialogues in theatre and cultural politics*. New York: Routledge, pp. 46–58.

Brahma, Jhana, Paravala, Vinod and Belavadi, Vasiki (2019) 'Driving social change through Forum Theatre: a study of Jana Sanskriti in West Bengal, India', *Asia Pacific Media Education*. Australia: University of Wollongong, pp. 1–14.

Chaudhuri, Prasun (2018) 'My *mitti*, my life and my death'. *The Telegraph*, Kolkata, 22 July, p. 17.

Cohen-Cruz, Jan and Schutzman, Mady (eds) (2006) *A Boal companion: dialogues in theatre and cultural politics*. New York: Routledge.

Da Costa, Dia (2007) 'Tensions of neo-liberal development: state discourse and dramatic oppositions in West Bengal', *Contributions to Indian Sociology*, 42(3), pp. 297–320.

Da Costa, Dia (2009) *Development dramas: reimagining rural political action in Eastern India*. New Delhi: Routledge.

Da Costa, Dia (2010a) 'Subjects of struggle: theatre as space of political economy', *Third World Quarterly*, 31(4), pp. 617–35.

Da Costa, Dia (ed.) (2010b) *Scripting power: Jana Sanskriti on and offstage*. Kokata: Camp.

Da Costa, Dia (2012) 'Learning from labour: the space and work of activist theatre', *Contemporary South Asia*, 20(1), pp. 119–33.

Diamond, David (2007) *Theatre for living: the art and science of community-based dialogue*. Victoria, Canada: Trafford.

Doat, Géraldine (2007) *Théâtre déclencheur: le Jana Sanskriti en Inde, arme de construction massive*. Grenoble: Université Stendhal Grenoble 3.

Freire, Paulo (1970) Pedagogy of the oppressed. New York: Herder and Herder.

Freire, Paulo (1998) *Pedagogy of freedom: ethics, democracy, and civic courage*. Lanham, MD: Rowman and Littlefield.

Fritz, Birgit (2012) *InExactArt: the autopoeietic theatre of Augusto Boal.* Translated by Lana Sendzimir and Ralph Yarrow. Stuttgart: Ibidem.

Fritz, Birgit (2016) *The courage to become: Augusto Boal's revolutionary politics of the body.* Translated by Lana Sendzimir and Ralph Yarrow. Vienna: Danzig & Unfried.

Fromm, Erich (1956) *The art of loving.* New York: Harper Row.

Frost, Anthony and Yarrow, Ralph (2015) *Improvisation in drama, theatre and performance: history, practice, theory.* Basingstoke: Palgrave.

Ganguly, Sanjoy (2009) *Where we stand: five plays by Sanjoy Ganguly.* Kolkata: Camp. Republished 2018; Kolkata: JSIRRI.

Ganguly, Sanjoy (2010) *Jana Sanskriti, Forum Theatre and democracy in India.* London: Routledge

Ganguly, Sanjoy (2017) *From Boal to Jana Sankriti: practice and principles.* London: Routledge.

Ganguly, Sanjoy (2019) lecture notes, unpublished draft

Ganguly, Sanjoy (2020) email to Ralph Yarrow, 21 January.

Hoff, Karla, Jalan, Jyotsna and Santra, Sattwik (2021) 'Theater of the Oppressed empowers women: evidence from India', forthcoming.

Howe, Kelly, Boal, Julian and Soeiro, José (eds) (2019) *The Routledge companion to Theatre of the Oppressed.* London & New York: Routledge.

Iyengar, Sameera (2001) 'Performing presence: Feminism and theatre in India', PhD thesis, University of Chicago.

Jelinek, Elfriede (1984) 'Was geschah nachdem Nora ihren Mann verlassen hatte', in *Theaterstücke.* Köln: Prometh.

Johnston, Chris (2005) *House of games.* London: Nick Hern.

Kahane, Adam (2010) *Power and love: a theory and practice of social change.* San Francisco: Berrett Koehler.

Kapadia, Karin (2012) 'Review of da Costa, *Dia, Development Dramas: Reimagining Rural Political Action in Eastern India*', *Progress in Development Studies*, 12(2&3), pp. 245–257.

Katyal, Anjum (1996) '"A coming together; an affirmation; a sharing". Kulavai: a report', *Seagull Theatre Quarterly*, 9, pp. 41–53.

Kompogiorgas, Sergio. (2019) 'Doll's House Jokering: a night to remember', email, March.

Lynne, Tamara (2014) 'Theatre as an act of transgression', *Perspectives on Anarchist Theory*, 27. Institute for Anarchist Studies.

Mohan (Da Costa), Dia (2008) 'From alienation to healthy culture: the particularity of Jana Sanskriti's use of "theatre of the oppressed" in rural Bengal, India', *Sanskriti* (an internet magazine published by Jana Sanskriti). Available at: www.janasanskriti.org.

Prendergast, Monica and Saxton, Juliana (eds) (2009) *Applied theatre: international case studies and challenges for practice*. Chicago: University of Chicago Press.

Poutot, Clément (2015) *Le theatre de l'opprimé: matrice symbolique de l'espace public*. Université de Caen Basse-Normandie: Thèse de Doctorat.

Schutzman, Mady and Cohen-Cruz, Jan (1994) *Playing Boal: theatre, therapy, activism*. Abingdon and New York: Routledge.

Srampickal, Joseph (1994) *Voice to the voiceless: the power of people's theatre in India*. New Delhi: Manohar.

Watson, Ian (2001) *Performer training: development across cultures*. Amsterdam: Harwood.

Yarrow, Ralph (2012) 'Performing agency: body learning, forum theatre and interactivity as democratic strategy', *Studies in South Asian Film and Media*, 4(2), pp. 211–26.

Yarrow, Ralph (2017) 'From performers to spectactivists: Jana Sanskriti's training for agency in and beyond theatre'. *Indian Theatre Journal*, 1(1), pp. 29–37.

INDEX

Note: **Bold** page numbers refer to key passages and accounts of plays.